DONE WITH DEMENTIA

Keeping your parents together

Linda McKendry

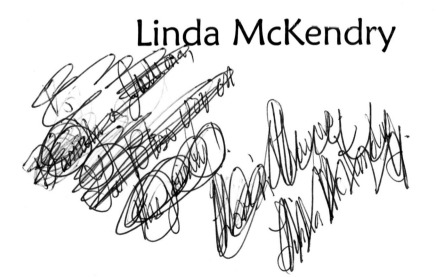

Done With Dementia

Copyright © 2020 by Linda McKendry

Printed in Canada

ISBN

978-0-2288-2222-6 (Hardcover)

978-0-2288-2223-3 (Paperback)

978-0-2288-2221-9 (eBook)

978-0-9781470-4-4 (Second Edition Printed in Canada)

DEDICATION

In Memory of John and Lydia Gamble

Our Precious Parents

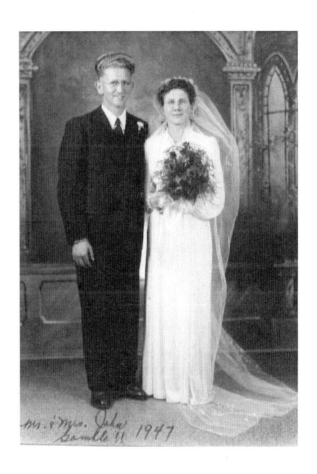

TABLE OF CONTENTS

ACKNOWLEDGEMENTS

My Guarantee: We ploughed through the journey of keeping our parents together and giving them the best care and comfort we could. We used the resources we had to the best of our ability or we found the resources we needed. We researched and applied professional and practical advice. You can learn from what we did to help you decide if you can or want to care for your parents and keep them together. You will be educated, motivated, inspired, and empowered to learn from all the "mistakes" we made.

Begging Forgiveness: I am begging forgiveness from my siblings and others who went on this journey with me if I do not remember the exact dates and times or tell the story differently than they remember it. Firstly, it's my story, and secondly, I know we all saw it in the light of our own circumstances and lifestyles.

A Prophetic Word: My involvement as primary caregiver for our parents fulfilled a prophetic word I gave to my Dad at age two, when he walked in the house and said, "Who's the boss in this house?" and I replied, "I is!" When they needed it, someone had to become the "boss" of the process and take the legal authority as Enduring Power of Attorney. I feel I was called and chosen by God for "such a time as this."

FOREWORD

Esther Susan "Susie" Unger (nee Gamble)

It was long ago and far away. In a remote, dusty region of India, 110 degrees in the shade, a little baby was born into a missionary family - the last of four children. Linda, the oldest, decided to christen this new arrival long before it was born. Long before the gender was even known! "Her name is going to be 'Susie'." The parents, John and Lydia called her Esther Susan, but "Susie" was the one that stuck. The bossy older sister was good at calling the shots!

It looks like Linda is still operating in that gift as she is asking little sister, Susie, to write the foreword for her new book. Of course, I am happy to do it as I have nothing but admiration and the greatest respect for my big sis.

Done With Dementia is birthed from years of taking the reins and assuming the responsibility of caring for our dear parents, John and Lydia, whose lives exemplified a great spirit of adventure, a genuine love for others, and a life well-lived!

The saying goes, "A foolish person learns from their own mistakes and a wise person learns from others." This book is about passing on what was learned as we traveled the road to dementia. The journey took a winding path, from occasional checking in, to 24/7 nonstop care.

As so often happens in these situations, Linda became the parent and our parents became like children. Under her compassionate nurturing care, Mom and Dad entered into their twilight years with a sense of security and comfort. The rest of us siblings came alongside as best we could. Together, with Linda at the helm, we kept a tender watch over them until they took their last breath, within 69 days of each other.

Words cannot express how much we owe Linda for all that she did for Mom and Dad, which was often under difficult personal circumstances.

I believe this book can offer crucial knowledge and insight to anyone who decides to navigate the odyssey of caring for parents with dementia. That expedition can be harrowing at times, but with adequate help and support, we can arrive at destination's end with a sense of personal satisfaction that we have honored our parents.

KEEPING YOUR PARENTS TOGETHER

INTRODUCTION
Plan While You Can

It's one thing for a couple who have been married for many years to be separated for a short time due to travel, work, or a temporary stay in a hospital when each knows and understands the situation. When one has dementia and can't remember why their mate isn't in their normal place, it causes all sorts of anxiety. It's like the first time a parent has to leave their child in someone else's care and the child is screaming as if the parent is deserting them for life and never coming back.

Our systems aren't designed to keep couples together unless they are functioning with reasonable mental clarity, regardless of physical disabilities or limitations. Couples who have been married for many years intuitively rely on each other for subtle, often unseen things that keep them confident and able to face each day. They know these nuances, gestures, tones of voice, glances, and special touch. Even familiar fragrances from their spouse bring comfort, whether it's a grooming product, or a liniment for sore joints.

It's not uncommon for a partner to die shortly after their mate passes away because such a big part of them is missing. Often a person with dementia will only listen to the one who's been advising, comforting, or even scolding for years. A mate can often have the best calming affect when someone is being asked to endure a treatment or attempt to learn something new.

How many of our love songs have the phrase, "lost without you…"? This is especially true of couples who have lived long lives and grown old together. It's not right to tear them apart for any reason, for any extended length of time and expect either of them to thrive. The element of dementia in one or both of them just adds to the confusion, causes conflicts, and diminishes a sense of well-being.

If You Wait, it Could be Too Late!

What Done-With-Dementia was for our family, and what it took to keep them together is what this book is all about. Left to the system, they would have been separated because they each needed different levels of care. This would have made it more difficult for us to visit them, and it would have cost a lot more. This is our story of committing to keep them together, and what we had to do to make that happen. Many visitors to their house, and strangers we encountered in restaurants and malls, would also ask us how we were managing. Someone suggested I should write a book. Someone else suggested I design a course. Therefore, this is that experience put into book form.

Yelling FORE!

On the golf course, you'll hear players yell, "Fore!" as a warning, there's a ball coming fast and you don't want to be in the way. Dementia doesn't give warning. In addition, it can come fast. It aims for the head, the memory, which affects mindful activities. I'm yelling "Fore!" to give you the warning.

FORE is the acronym I use to identify the four main issues in dealing with dementia. When I began to write this book, I knew that the very first word was "familiarity" when it comes to dealing with dementia. I thought, "What do I have to advise people to look for or do before they can even contemplate caring for their parents to keep them together?" In that word, "before" are four things to do for yourself and your parents.

• Familiarity. Keeping as many things familiar for your parents is the key. Since the main symptom of dementia is memory loss, this is the best thing you can do for them. Begin today to observe the things that are familiar in your parent's lives. As an adult, you have probably moved away a long time ago and what you remember as being familiar may have changed. (See Research Options p.33 and the Survey Chapter p.236)

• Organization. Everything you organize for them is easier when you keep the familiar things and people in mind. Organize the tangible, practical things as well as the activities and events around what is familiar to them. I will give many illustrations and stories of how we did this for Mom and Dad. If dementia hasn't invaded their lives look for changes to organizing their space or their time to help prepare them for downsizing or moving.

• Routines: When you know your parents' routines that have become habitual as they manage their days, weeks, and months it is easier to make them comfortable, happy, and safe when the time comes to help them. What they have done habitually requires less memory. Extreme dementia can negate their mental capacities, so routines then are more important for the caregivers' schedules and assignments.

• EPOA: This stands for Enduring Power of Attorney and it is the last in the list, but not the least. Have a trusted friend, or family member legally assigned to handle their affairs. To the degree that they are reluctant to let someone find out what they need, their EPOA should be someone with whom they are familiar. However, this is critical to be dealt with before dementia symptoms make it legally impossible for them to sign off.

WHEN DEMENTIA STRIKES

Stuff We Didn't Know or Even Look At

SIGNS

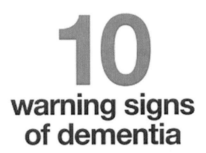

Dementia is not a part of normal ageing.
Talk to a doctor or contact the
Alzheimer association in your country.

Alzheimer's Disease
International
The global voice on dementia

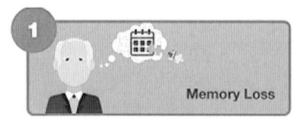

Everyone wants to know what the Warning Signs of Dementia are. This one is published by the Alzheimer's Disease International and I want to share with you how we knew that some of these signs were affecting our parent's sanity and safety. Look for the signs to verify if dementia is surfacing.

In the case of our parents, if you asked Mom, she would say, "I don't know", if she didn't remember. If she gave you an answer it was usually because she really did remember. She was also fond of saying, "Ask your Dad."

If you asked Dad, he would confidently tell you something that you would eventually find out wasn't a fact. That made Mom easier to work with and Dad always a little suspect. We had to check into his responses more often.

You may have to check into their answers if you suspect dementia to verify whether they remember or not. The more time you spend with them and become familiar with their lives, the better you can tell if their memory is compromised due to dementia.

Everyone has memory loss. You know that "it's on the tip of my tongue..." kind of fact that you've temporarily forgotten, but not really. You know that you can't remember. Mom and Dad's gerontologist told me once that what causes the most memory loss when it's not dementia is mental overload; i.e. multi-tasking or trying to think of too many things at one time. She confirmed that making lists, having systems in place, documenting important information and events is a mentally healthy thing to do.

Linda McKendry

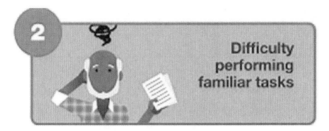

No one wants to forget important things.

When Dad had to point out to us that he had found the eggs in Mom's dresser drawer instead of in the frying pan, we knew there was a problem. We asked if this was happening a lot or just that once. He couldn't answer. He was teasing her about laying her eggs in the drawer and trying to make light of it.

Shortly after that, he invited us over to have breakfast with them at the house. When I went into the kitchen to see if I could help, the muffins were in the oven in a plastic blister pack and the cinnamon buns in the foil pan in the microwave.

I checked with him to see if he realized his mistake getting them mixed up and he just laughed at what he had done and asked me to switch them up. The oven wasn't turned on, so that was a relief. It also showed us that he was trying to take over from what Mom had typically done. Mom seemed oblivious to it all.

This was just another eye-opener and it made me decide to come by more often and check into what was happening in the kitchen and with meal preparation. That was when I found out that they were getting Meals on Wheels twice a week. But they were also rationing them by only eating half at one sitting and often forgetting what was still in the toaster oven or microwave.

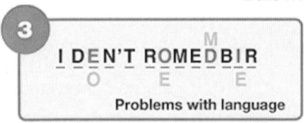

Problems with language

This warning sign is both evident in writing and speaking. However, my Mother was really funny as she would often say,

"I'm getting my merds all wixed." She and her sister, my Aunt Ruthie, had fairy tales memorized and would entertain us for hours with them. My favorite was "Pinderella and the Cince" and the "Gairy Fodmother."

So I have to say that I don't remember any problems with having trouble getting words out. I would have to ask other caregivers if they recall issues with understanding what Mom or Dad were saying due to their dementia. Their replies were usually logical.

Mom did stop writing in her diary and sending out notes and cards, which she loved to do, but I can't tell you when that was without going through her journals and diaries. One thing that really upset her was when her good old typewriter was replaced with a word processor and then a laptop.

Her frustration with those grew to the point where she just gave up and didn't want to write any more. Dad had study notes for their home group and Bible classes he taught and I used to type them up for him and print them out for his students each week. This is what Mom had done before.

I believe I would have picked up on this warning sign if it had been obvious. Dad did write really tiny and we used to tease him about writing like a doctor making out a prescription that was hard to read. This was never a real warning sign for me, but since I have dyslexia, it may seem like a sign in me!

19

Linda McKendry

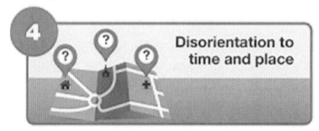

This warning sign was hinted at when Mom and Dad drove to a convention. Dad shared that each day they had gotten lost from the hotel to the event. He was kind of blaming Mom for not navigating correctly as the map reader. He said that for some reason they always went out from the hotel the wrong way.

When you ask me or my siblings what was the first time they realized Mom or Dad might have dementia we all point to the same event. Mom would walk a couple of blocks to do a little grocery shopping, visit their pharmacist and the hearing aid clinic. One day as she came home she suddenly didn't know where she was or how to get home.

A panic led her to say a prayer and next thing she knew she was at the house. She was so upset that she stumbled through the back door and burst out crying. Dad was in his clock shop with a customer and came up to lead her into their bedroom to rest until he was free to find out what had happened and comfort her.

The day Dad lost his driver's license was when he didn't show up for a program. Thank God he had his cell phone with him so I could call. He was sitting in the emergency waiting room at a hospital. I asked him to let me talk to one of the nurses and she told me where he was. He even had the name of the hospital wrong.

It was a sad day because Dad loved to drive. Mechanically he could drive okay, but his mind couldn't keep his location clear or the directions to take.

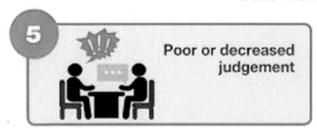

To me this means an inability to judge correctly or make a decision based on a good reason. The example that comes to mind is how much we depended on Dad to pick up the slack for Mom's dementia. It was a whole lot later that we realized he didn't have the ability and it was very stressful for him.

One example is when they were in the Assisted Living facility. Dad called and asked if I would "keep Lydia" for a while at my office while he did some shopping. My office was in a central commercial location and I didn't have any appointments so I said, "Of course."

It was early spring. Snow was still on the ground but a lot of ground and pavement was showing through. When Dad brought Mom in, I was shocked to see she was wearing light cotton blouse and skirt. She had sandals on and no coat. I was even more shocked that she didn't seem to notice her feet were getting wet from the puddles.

When I confronted Dad about her lack of a coat and boots, he said, "I don't dress your Mummy. She dresses herself." And that was that.

However, when I found out that Dad was getting a perm for Mom every two weeks so he could go out for a couple of hours on his own, it was one of the 'last straws' to realizing that neither of them was operating with good judgement for themselves or for each other. I began to see the desperate need for change.

Linda McKendry

Problems keeping track of things

When you read my book, Done-With-Dementia you will notice how many times I use the word 'familiar'. When items are put into 'familiar' places they don't get lost … that is IF you can remember where those places are.

We had one occasion at their home when everyone was looking for some e-tickets and a travel schedule. Dad was pressuring Mom to look in a few more places, kind of blaming her and had the rest of us looking also.

At one point I looked over at the pile of papers and books stacked beside his easy chair and decided to go through them. I sat in the chair and one by one put each book and paper on my lap. Sure enough, right at the bottom was what we were looking for. It was obvious that Mom wouldn't have put them there. Dad didn't own up to it either.

We made a huge effort to put the furnishings they were used to in the places they were moved to at the Lodge. I presumed that they would automatically look in a specific drawer for socks and underwear without even thinking. But as much as we were able to keep a lot of their familiar things, it was still all rearranged and in a different atmosphere, so they found it hard to find things.

One time I used the washroom in their unit and Mom had used her pull-ups to line the waste basket instead of a recycled grocery bag. More and more 'little' things were adding up to make me look at better living and caregiving options for them.

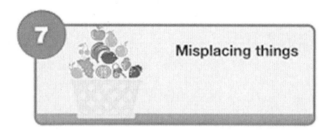

7 Misplacing things

There are only two reasons why things get misplaced. First, there wasn't a conscious decision to make a 'home' for specific items. Second, if there was, it can't be remembered. I misplace things frequently when I haven't taken the time to decide on where something is going to be stored when not in use.

We all know what it is like to 'trace our steps' so we go back and find something that was set down mindlessly and forgotten. Or ask, "Has anyone seen my__?"

Mom and Dad always kept certain things in spots where even us kids knew where to find them. The house was well organized in a logical way. The problem began when we were out. Mom would leave her purse or her cane somewhere. Dad would leave his hat.

Once we realized that Mom would forget her purse if someone didn't lengthen the strap and put it over her shoulder, we kept it at home. Identity theft was the main risk and as long as she had a tissue in her pocket she didn't seem to need or want anything else.

They never did adapt to the facility and were looking for things that we had sold, given away, or disposed of in the downsizing.

It was sad to keep having to tell them what had happened to specific items. They would ask again and again.

Dad always wanted to know where his lathe was from his clock shop. Mom didn't ask about anything except if Dad was gone for an extended time. "Where's my Johnny?"

23

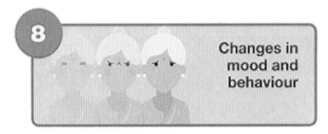

8 Changes in mood and behaviour

Both of them exhibited changes in mood and behavior. Dad was better at hiding his feelings except when pressuring Mom. He expected things from her that she no longer did or was capable of. He'd ask for help with the laundry but not say it was because Mom couldn't.

Mom would frequently sit and cry all day and when asked why she was crying, she would act as if she didn't know why! Her mood could change in an instant, especially if one of the caregivers who weren't family came in the room.

It was totally uncharacteristic of her to be rude or mean, but she lashed out at the nurses and often told them they were "Stupid." Or, "I don't like you." We credited some of this change to when Dad came home from his surgery and needed a lot of extra care from the nurses. Mom would see them changing his ileostomy bag or helping him bathe.

When she came closer to see, Dad would shoo her away, which probably made her even more upset. We were constantly challenged with keeping her happy and content. The magic was in playing Gaither Gospel music DVDs or her favorite classic movies. Her expression would change and she would be clapping or singing right along.

We also limited Dad's watching the news when she was in the living room since there was so much violence and bad reports that she would react as if she could talk to the TV and they would hear what she was saying.

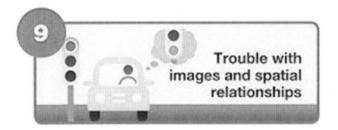

The example given here has to do with driving and I already covered Dad's issues with that. One thing about our parents is that they were amazingly mobile and healthy for their age when they weren't suffering a temporary crisis.

We were aware of and trained to hold a firm but gentle grip on an elbow and walk close to steer and point out obstacles like steps and curbs. Many seniors have falls because they are reaching out to what they believe is a stable object and it isn't.

We were shown by the Occupational Therapist to remind Dad to back into a chair and reach down for the arms to settle himself in it. He forgot this once and in heading to the chair and reaching down to the arm, his hand slipped off; he fell forward and fractured some ribs when he landed on it with full force.

It wasn't until the next morning when he couldn't raise himself in bed to get up that he confessed what had happened. We took him to the doctor for x-rays and pain medication.

In case you are wondering, I used his leather belt attached to the foot board for him to pull on as I lifted him! He backed into chairs from that day on. Sometimes Mom would comment about the trees at the rental house and tell us she remembered them being planted. I don't think that had much to do with "images or spatial relationships". It was, after all, a real tree and it triggered a real memory.

Linda McKendry

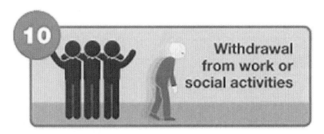

This is an interesting warning sign. Dad was leading a home group and teaching Sunday School right up until they moved into the Assisted Living facility. Because he had conducted services at the chapel in this facility and three of their friends in the same parish lived there, we assumed they would make friends and minister in a similar way.

While they were seen regularly in the common room for the snack times and some of the special entertainment, they weren't associating with anyone there. As far as we knew they were driving themselves to church each Sunday and engaging with all their friends and acquaintances there.

I wasn't as involved at that point and we were taking a lot for granted because on the surface and in passing most things seemed like they would work their way out.

Other residents began to share with me that often Mom was sitting on a chair outside the elevator door crying because Dad had sent her to their room after a meal and she didn't know where to go. They would go and find him and let him know. I personally believe that he began to feel embarrassed about her behavior and socialized less and less.

On the other hand, the residents also told me that every evening after dinner they could be seen walking hand in hand out around the grounds and they all thought it was so 'cute'.

Mom was usually happy to see anyone who was giving her attention, except for the foreign nurses, which we never totally understood.

CONCLUSION

There are dozens of levels and types of dementia. Many of these Warning Signs become very severe and extreme. We witnessed seniors with dementia being medicated to the point where they seemed to be barely living. Our foreign worker nurses disclosed some of the things they had to do to people in their care at lockdown facilities because of outbursts of violence or wandering. I believe that because there are so many patients in some facilities being looked after by a limited number of people the risks have to be reduced to prevent harm to anyone.

We kept our parents together and cared for them with the help of good medical professional advice and 24/7 supervision. We gave them more of the one-on-one care and attention that prevented them from becoming agitated over things that were never an issue for us. In the Assisted Living they had witnessed one lady throwing her hot soup in the lap of her table mate. Meals in their own home were always more pleasant and full of fun. After we moved them out of the facility there were many days when four generations met for lunch or supper since my daughter and her children lived a block away.

We also believe we had the mercy and grace of God since we are a family of faith. Prayer was in our daily routine which gave us a lot of peace and calm. A lot can be Done-With-Dementia. It isn't hopeless and because they had a long marriage and the most familiar thing in their lives was each other. Being together was one of the forces that kept them happier and heathier all around. No regrets!

STATISTICS

Here are some of the projected statistics in charts you may find interesting.

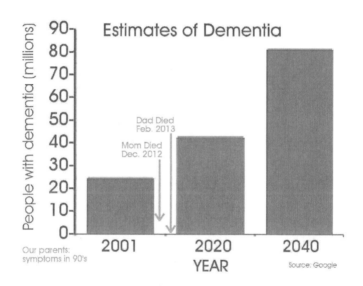

As of the publishing date of this book, we are on the later years of these charts. Our parents were in their seventies when we first noticed any dementia (1992). By the time they passed away, they were in their nineties (2012 and 2013). You can see the increase in dementia cases as the years go by and people get older.

I don't know if we had looked at the statistics on dementia if we would have done anything different. We saw that our parents needed help. We loved them. We remembered all the sacrifices they had made for us. We recognized that they had to change our diapers when we were little, so some of what we accepted to do for their care came naturally. Without question. It wasn't a matter of if because of our promise to them, but more of how to make it work.

Linda McKendry

PREVALENCE OF ALZHEIMER'S DISEASE
(BY DECADES IN U.S.A. FROM 1900-2060

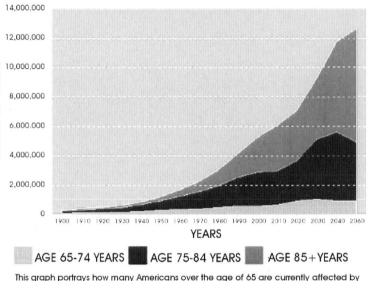

AGE 65-74 YEARS ■ AGE 75-84 YEARS ■ AGE 85+YEARS

This graph portrays how many Americans over the age of 65 are currently affected by Alzheimer's, and a projection of how many more will become affected with it as time passes.
w3.ouhsc.edu

In our lives and Dad's church we saw old people suffering from weaknesses, infirmities, and senility due to old age. The news was full of reports of this condition named "Alzheimer's" where people forgot a lot. There were even jokes and humorous cartoons which in any society is a coping mechanism to help deal with the difficult. I had visited the senior shut-ins with my pastor Dad many times, especially when I wanted to borrow the car while he was on call. I saw how much attention and care he gave to them in their homes, in hospitals or senior facilities.

We did discuss news reports of people in care facilities being abused and my sister was adamant that our parents would never be in a place where that would be risked. This was one of her big motives in wanting to personally take care of our parents. She and her husband talked for years of the dream home or duplex with Mom and Dad living next door. She was also the "baby" in the family and talked to Mom almost every day. She was like an only child because we, the older siblings, were sent to an international boarding school in northern India and she was raised without us around in her pre-school years. She was passionate about their care.

We were so focused on them as our parents. We always saw them as one unit because they did so many things together. We didn't stop to look at the statistics. We didn't follow anyone's story. I believe that the only difference it would have made was to convince us even more that to keep them together, we needed very special care that isn't typically offered in the mainstream. Getting old is something we all face, and we were the children, the next generation. We didn't see ourselves as being too old, or unable, to care for our parents. Most of us were already grandparents or didn't have our adult children still at home.

We were raised to believe in the Ten Commandments given to Moses in the Bible, including the one, "Honor thy father and thy mother: that thy days may be long upon the land which the LORD thy God giveth thee." On a humorous note, I used to think my days would have to be "long" upon the land, so I could out-live them and have my life back! Short of a miracle, you know the end will be death and then they and you really are Done-With-Dementia.

Now that I am telling our story and sharing some ideas on what can be Done-With-Dementia, I know I have to present the current statistics because the need is even greater now. The costs are going up. The level of care is going down unless you have the financial resources to pay for personal 24/7 care. The facilities that accommodate couples, regardless of their level of required care, are few and still far between. This means that there is still the reality of parents being cared for by their family (mostly daughters) as one of the available options.

Just My Opinion

We institutionalize our preschool children in day care homes and public schools and put our aging parents in old age homes for the sake of our independence and convenience. After looking after our parents, we would recommend it to anyone. For us it wasn't something we tried. We just did it. We had some terrible days and nights, and some great ones. By the time we felt burnout and wanted to quit, we checked out the options and concluded we were already in the best place possible. We learned to give ourselves a break. We asked for help. We prayed a lot and we changed our attitude and heart. God helped. He gave strength, wisdom, and favor. Our joy returned as we continued the journey.

Love is the answer.

RESEARCH OPTIONS

PLAN WHILE YOU CAN

LEGAL

I am an associate for an organization that specializes in prepaid legal plans. At our first family meeting with Mom and Dad to discuss their plans for their aging, I offered to become their Enduring Power of Attorney (EPOA) with my brother authorized to take over if I couldn't or didn't want to. We both lived in the same city as Mom and Dad, while our other siblings lived further away. We also updated their wills and their personal directives (i.e. living will) which outlined their preferences for emergency care under specific circumstances.

While I knew the power and authority that came with this, I was advised by the lawyer the responsibility. She gave me one important piece of advice. She said, "Always confer with your siblings when you have decisions to make on your parent's behalf. Report to them regularly. Get their opinions and take them into consideration. However, the final say or action you take will be legally yours. The courts don't take lightly to abuse or misuse of this privilege." Most of the time it was easy to make decisions on their behalf because logic and love were guiding forces. When it was hard, I would gather opinions and preferences from my siblings and then decide.

Linda McKendry

My siblings will confess that what they liked most was that someone they trusted was making the mundane, daily decisions. They will also confess that there were times when they questioned my wisdom, but in the end realized I had limitations and couldn't control everything.

Question: Do your parents have their wills, personal directives, and EPOA in place? Don't wait.

The will is important to have in place for many reasons, but it also has more to do with after they die and our main concern was what to do while they were still alive. If you aren't an heir, or the executor, this won't concern you at all.

The personal directive, which is done with the help of their physicians, is important to have in your "back pocket". In case of emergency the EMS need to know what treatment to give and what level of life support is requested depending on the situation. This also may never be activated. Research information on getting them a Life Capsule for EMS that goes in the freezer. A neon EMS Alert sticker goes on the fridge door. This capsule contains their life support choices endorsed by their doctor, and a list of their medications and any medical conditions to note, like diabetes.

The most important document for you to acquire is the EPOA, or Enduring Power of Attorney. This is what gives you the authority to act on their behalf and it is very serious. It can be taken advantage of, so the courts do not look lightly on anyone who deceives seniors or takes advantage of the elderly. Family or not.

So...

1.   Do they have their wills, personal directives, and EPOA in place?

- Yes? Should it stay the same? Be someone younger? Someone living closer to them? Someone who better understands their needs?
- No? Make it a priority. If you have a mind to, offer to become their EPOA. This doesn't mean you will automatically be caring for them, but you can have a lot of say in it.

2.   Are they mentally fit to meet with a lawyer and sign off on their will, personal directive, and EPOA?

- Yes? Do this immediately. Do not put it off.
- No? Contact their lawyer as a matter of interest as a "next of kin" and find out what legal rights you do have on their behalf. It can be court appointed.
- You can still do a lot to influence their care.
- You will still be respected and recognized by those in authority when decisions need to be made.

You are welcome to check out this direct link to my

LegalShield website: https://lindamckendry.wearelegalshield.com/

Here you can access the services of legal counsel for many typical life issues. I used LegalShield many times over the twenty years we took on this responsibility. They did the conveyance on the sale of their house. We also used LegalShield for immigration law and hiring our foreign workers.

The level of legal authority as an EPOA covers authority and responsibility for taking care of your parent's finances. It's never too soon to show an interest for the purpose of helping them make decisions in line with their plans and preferences. Finances affect every aspect of our lives and definitely extended care and lifestyles. Here are some questions to help you get started, hopefully, with their approval and help:

- What resources are available for them right now?
- What investments or retirement savings do they have?
- What benefits, programs, pensions, or other support is available for them? (e.g. Veterans) Check out government and financial assistance based on:
- Joint Income
- Age/Status as Seniors
- Referrals and Prescriptions

While you may have missed the legal stuff until now, as long as you make decisions in a logical and loving way, you will likely be on a good path.

You can still help them investigate other things they need for their current care and comfort. Legally you can't get their personal information, unless they choose to trust you and give you all the facts. However, as their loved one, no one can stop you from helping them plan. You can get a lot of information about facilities, programs, support, and other's experiences.

LOGICAL

So many of the things you can do are just logical or common sense. In terms of the priorities, what they need the most that requires the greatest attention to time and detail will be at the top of your list. During a medical crisis, everything comes to a stop while you call 911 and wait for the EMS. During recovery, temporary treatments and medications are monitored more closely so that becomes a priority to document and record.

Depending on the number of people assisting in their care around the clock, systems need to be in place for communicating from shift to shift, like they would do in a commercial facility or a hospital. This is where calendars, log books, white boards, lists of contacts, and schedules with activities are tools to add to everyone's comfort in the process. (See Chapter: Making Everything Work.)

Knowing your parent's routines, habits, and preferences makes logical placement of their possessions and meal planning easier for everyone. To the degree they are still able to do things for themselves, such as grooming or dressing with some or no help, use logic to make it safer and easier for them. You will see the details of what we did in our story.

The fine line is between letting some things go completely, or a little longer between servicing, and letting things go too long so the work is more difficult. Laundry, for example, doesn't have to be done as often when there are plenty of socks, underwear, shirts, sheets and towels. It's more efficient and economical to do a larger load less often than frequent smaller ones. This allows you to take home laundry and add it to your own without creating any panic over a week or two.

Logic and common sense will help you get creative with what the needs are to keep your parents together in their own home. If they have savings or a "nest egg" this is what it is for! Be frugal and efficient. Save time and money wherever you can, but also be prepared to invest where it will make their quality of life comfortable and safe.

Linda McKendry

FACILITIES – YOUR PARENTS' OPTIONS

There are different levels of care and facilities. Some are designed to handle all levels of care in a single complex. Most specialize in just one level of care.

TAKE NOTE: Senior facilities are businesses. Slick ads, attractive websites, and promotional materials are all designed for investors and for attracting residents or patients. Some are associated with the system for the purpose of making sure no one in society is neglected. But it's all based on what you can afford. I'm not against these places and I've been privileged to entertain in many of them and get to know the staff and residents. Most staff are doing the best they can for their employers, the residents, and visiting family and friends.

Facilities cost money for furnishing and maintenance. Staff are hired. Programs are sponsored. Meals are prepared and served. Care, comfort, and safety all require investments of time and money. They have to be run in a professional, business-like manner.

My Advice?

- Check online.
- Arrange tours.
- Visit with residents.
- Talk to others.
- Look closely.

And, most of all don't be afraid to take your parents out of a facility if it's not working. Move them back to their own home, if possible, or find another place more suitable for you and for them like we did.

Done With Dementia

Here is a chart and I'll list some of the pros and cons below it.

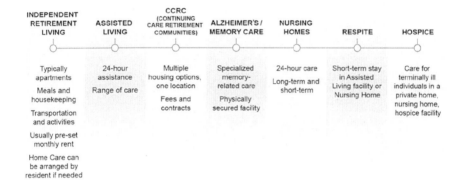

INDEPENDENT RETIREMENT LIVING	ASSISTED LIVING	CCRC (CONTINUING CARE RETIREMENT COMMUNITIES)	ALZHEIMER'S / MEMORY CARE	NURSING HOMES	RESPITE	HOSPICE
Typically apartments	24-hour assistance	Multiple housing options, one location	Specialized memory-related care	24-hour care	Short-term stay in Assisted Living facility or Nursing Home	Care for terminally ill individuals in a private home, nursing home, hospice facility
Meals and housekeeping	Range of care	Fees and contracts	Physically secured facility	Long-term and short-term		
Transportation and activities						
Usually pre-set monthly rent						
Home Care can be arranged by resident if needed						

Retirement Facilities:

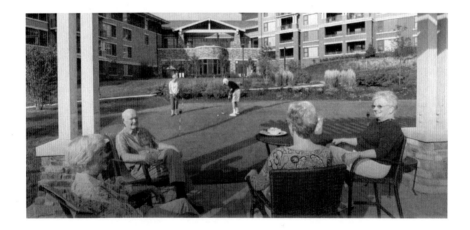

Also called "Independent Retirement Living" is for people who want some amenities along with meals, housekeeping, and no maintenance. Some units have kitchens and garages as part of a larger complex with options to eat at a communal dining room.

Linda McKendry

These are for people single or married who want to lead active lives with lots of social encounters, in-house programs, and ways to make their retirement more leisurely. Costs vary so it's worth checking into especially if your parents are frustrated or wearing themselves out with maintaining their own properties.

Assisted Living:

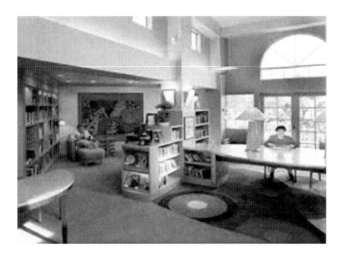

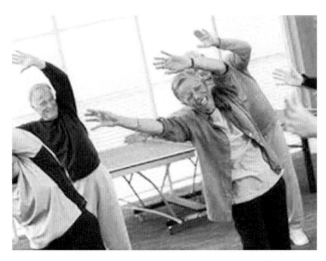

This level of care usually doesn't have suites or apartments, but studio rooms with a private bath and room enough for a single bed and small-scale furnishings. The residents can take advantage of the amenities and meals eaten in the common dining room. The rooms are equipped with emergency pull chains and two-way intercoms. The facility often has a nurse on staff and "home care" types of services are available for a fee. The downside is that the meals are scheduled and it's during this time that if a resident hasn't formally signed out the staff will come looking for them. It can also be frustrating if your parents are still driving, are out somewhere enjoying themselves, having a bite to eat, and not ready to rush back at the prescribed hour.

Extended Care:

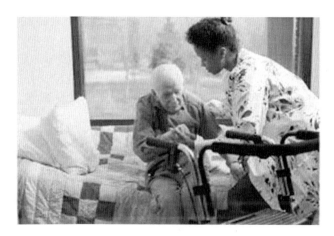

This facility accommodates residents for the rest of their life, unless they are hospitalized for something serious, or transferred to a hospice when terminal. Sometimes this is also referred to as a "Nursing Home". There is round-the-clock professional staff trained or experienced in caring for people with serious, chronic conditions. Modern monitoring equipment allows staff to care for multiple patients at one time. Facilities specializing in dementia and Alzheimer's have units that restrict outside access with special doors, alarms, and security systems.

Respite Care: This facility takes people in temporarily to either give the primary caregiver a break, or to strengthen a senior with therapy.

Hospices: These facilities specialize in taking care of people with terminal conditions. Palliative care is usually administered, and the rooms are designed to make visiting family and friends comfortable 24/7. The staff are highly trained or experienced in being with people when they pass and know how to make them comfortable. Palliative care at home means that the family or friends are responsible for administering the medications. Not everyone is comfortable doing that. In the hospice, or hospital, all the monitoring equipment is there too.

Home Care:

This is the main option that most seniors want. Most want to stay in their own home surrounded by the things that are familiar with the routine they are used to. They can eat what they want, when they want, and not have to go down miles of hallway to get to their rooms, or wait for available staff member to assist, or wait with dozens of others to use an elevator.

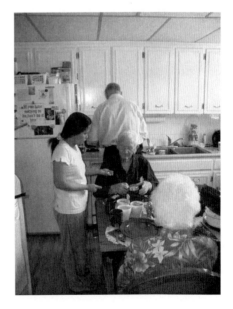

Done With Dementia

Most governments and communities prefer to subsidize home care and keep seniors in their own home which is why a lot of programs exist for different requirements. Where we live there is Aids to Daily Living that will pay to have safety items installed such as rails in halls and showers, raised toilet seats, and tub grab bars. Some of them provide the right type of walker, wheelchair, or portable potty close to a bed or chair. They often ask that these be donated to the Red Cross when no longer required.

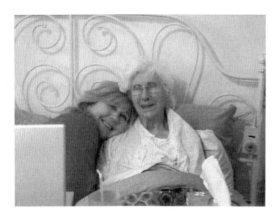 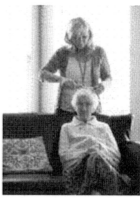

It isn't so much a matter of if they are going to have home care, but where. And it boils down to only three places.

- Theirs: Staying in their own home is always a preferred option for obvious reasons. If they aren't safe to be left alone then 24/7 supervision is required. Safety, sanitary, and maintenance issues must also be addressed.
- Yours: Your home may be the next most familiar place for them and at the very least you are there to supervise part time if not full time. You can still take advantage of available services and assistance since it's your parents and the condition of the house that qualify for the safety and comfort.

- <u>Others</u>: This is what we did when we took Mom and Dad out of Assisted Living and found a house to rent for them to live in. All the same services and assistance were made available. We did have to get written permission from the landlord for the Aids to Daily Living installation of rails and grab bars, but that was no problem.

In the case of their home or your own, if the mortgage is paid, the expenses are even less since there's no "rent" to pay. In our case, Self Managed Care Funding had nothing to do with the house and everything to do with hiring care. You could use a small portion of the funds to advertise the positions based on the assessment of the Home Care people in terms of the wage offered and the job description. You couldn't hire from the same agencies that Health Services used. Hiring foreign workers was another option we investigated. We found them diligent, hardworking, and motivated to integrate into the culture.

I once looked at the two seniors' facilities closer to my home in Calgary. One was more of a retirement center, so it wasn't suitable. The other had some in-house medical staff and a low level of dementia care but no adjoining rooms. The day I visited, it was dark, dingy, and had an atmosphere of doom and gloom. It was all decorated in shades of grey and blue with very dim lighting. My first thought was that they were taking advantage of the sky lights to save electricity, and it was a cloudy day.

So, it wasn't just the overall ambiance, but the convenience. Even though I would be able to walk to this center, there were more cons than pros compared to what we had set up, which was twenty minutes away from my home. A major move and another transition didn't make sense. Because of the dementia they were both manifesting, it would just create confusion for all of us and especially for them.

If you have done the research of commercial facility costs, you will realize the small amount of spending to secure some services ongoing to give everyone peace of mind. Technology has also provided some devices and services, such as GPS, remote surveillance, locking systems, monitors, alarms, and more, depending on the needs.

RECOMMENDATIONS
Go to Others

When you are looking at options of care for your parents to keep them together, you will often find yourself listening to other's experiences, as caregivers, or dementia care professionals. Ask the questions that concern you and listen to the answers that will help you make good decisions.

Ask questions and listen to the stories of adult children who have experience. Ask if they were happy with the care of their parents and if not find out why. Take their advice seriously but also research more than one case to avoid that single biased opinion.

Dementia care professionals, both working in facilities and involved in home care, can summarize pros and cons of each. Research multiple positions and remember that sometimes you get the most honest opinions from those who work behind the scenes in facilities.

Ask direct questions and pay attention to the attitude expressed. Watch the actions if you are observing care. Be fair in evaluating motives. Sometimes there are more issues than what is explained

Linda McKendry

or evident. The general list of needs, such as in my "M & M" list, are the same for most people regardless of the facility. (p.167)

LOVING

When all else fails there's always the loving thing to do. This is the motive to begin with and it comes with the honor and respect your parents are due, even if they haven't been ideal parents or you disagree with some of their ideologies. Each parent will tell you that they did the best they could with what they knew when you were born. If you are the oldest, like me, they cut their teeth on you and the others had a much easier time!

Anything about anybody can be irritating, annoying, and frustrating. It takes a lot of patience to live with another human being and often it means "submitting one to another in love". Love also demands doing hard things and things that might be uncomfortable temporarily. When your parent has a fall, fractures bones or bruises limbs, it's a painful process to help with recovery. When a technician is trying to get your parent to lie in an uncomfortable position to get a good x-ray you are there to help make it happen as quickly as possible. Dementia often makes these normal medical procedures seem like torture to the person who doesn't understand what is going on or why it is necessary.

There will be lots of temptations to get angry, be mean, or scold as if you are dealing with a naughty child, but love will come to the rescue. Someone with dementia will often forget the offense a few seconds after it happens, or they may decide for some strange reason to hold it against you ongoing. You won't know. But it's okay to say sorry. Say sorry for the situation. Say sorry for yourself and your own well-being and reach out in love no matter what.

Both my sister and I found that when we cupped my mother's face in our hands, looked her straight in the eyes, smiled and said, "I love you!" she would smile, say, "I love you too!" Then I would say, "I love you three!" And more often than not, she would say, "I love you four." And when she did, I knew a logical part of her was still there. Love is a decision. We love our children no matter how frustrated they make us because they are our children. We love our parents for the same reason and when we are called on to parent them, we love them even more.

FEEDBACK

Go to Your Parents

If your parents are well enough mentally to respond to the options you have found for them, plan a good time to approach them and share it. If it is only your decision or your family's, then orchestrate that meeting as soon as possible. Remember, even if they don't need these services yet, everyone knows availability, costs, and conditions for application. It's very comforting.

Share your research with your parents with love and concern for their care and without any pressure unless it's urgent. Don't overwhelm them with too much information at once. Short-list the options and give more details as they request them. Avoid confusion by not mentioning options that aren't feasible.

Gauge their comfort level and give them time to process, especially if they are still making good decisions for themselves daily. If you are just putting information out for the family in preparation for a key decision time, then leave it at that. No pressure. Some things may change if enough time passes.

Linda McKendry

Feel free to make documents, lists, and provide everyone with a little info packet if that suits you. Be sensitive to overload and resistance from siblings who may feel intimidated or guilty for not taking things more seriously themselves. Do everything with love, compassion, and patience.

PUTTING ALL OF THESE THINGS TOGETHER

Researching these options for your parents gives you the information you need. Armed with facts or valuable opinions you can confidently offer the help where it's needed the most.

A lot can be Done-With-Dementia!

BE THE HERO IN YOUR FAMILY

START TODAY

OUR STORY

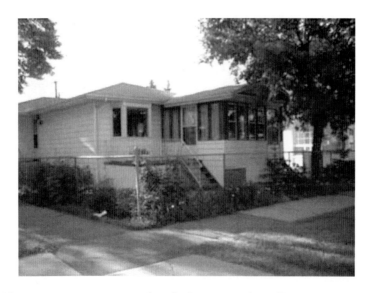

In 1992 our parents were in their seventies. Some symptoms of dementia had surfaced. We had a family meeting to let them share their thoughts and feelings about their future as they aged.

I was involved at that time with providing pre-paid legal plans which included preparation of wills, personal directives, and appointing powers of attorney. I understood the importance of having these documents up-to-date; including assigning trusted Enduring Powers of Attorney (EPOA). I offered to put that in place with the blessing of my parents and siblings. It represented a lot of authority and responsibility, but we were ready for any crisis.

We downsized and in 2007 moved them into an Assisted Living Facility with the promise that if it didn't work out in six months, we would move them back into their own home. We got to know a

Linda McKendry

lot about them between 1992 and the last day in their own home in 2007. Crisis had revealed more dementia and we were able to step in quickly. But this also showed us the areas in which they needed more help. I deliberately began to involve myself more in their lives and routines, including, going with them to appointments to meet the people with whom they were familiar.

It turned out to be a twenty year journey that I'm happy to share in hopes that it gives hope and help to those wanting to give care as children, or receive care as parents. The two major turning points were helping them into Assisted Living and then taking them out only seven months later. Therefore we show you what their lives were like before, during and after the Lodge.

BEFORE THE LODGE

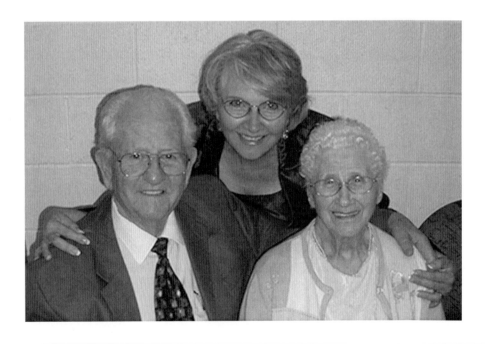

Following My Tears

An ounce of prevention… is worth a pound of tears. I sat in the boarding lounge at the Calgary Airport waiting for the flight that would move us to Toronto. I was leaving my parents and my children to follow my husband's corporate transfer. It was an amazing opportunity for him but my heart was breaking.

My daughter Kim, a newlywed, was the first to come for a visit. When I told her I had cried all the way to Toronto, she gave me a hug and said, "And I followed your little tears!"

Twelve years later I was sitting in the same airport waiting lounge crying again. This was our last flight before moving back to Alberta. I had just called my mother, who was not well, to say goodbye again and see how she was doing. It hit me. What if she dies! Those tears brought a prayer to my heart and I begged God, "Please don't let her die until we move back here so I can look after her." Little did I know how that prayer would be answered and what kind of responsibility I would take on.

I am a strong woman. My symbol is a swan. Gliding along on the surface like everything is under control and paddling like crazy underneath! I don't cry often. I figure it out, get grateful and positive, and carry on. But I've come to understand that when the tears do flow, it's a sign to follow them.

I closed a successful consulting business after eighteen years in July 2009 to care for my parents full time. My career success was due to figuring out ways to "educate, motivate, inspire, and entertain" audiences in the Science and Art of Merchandising and Display. Everything I taught was logical. I just created memorable ways to remember the main principles and rules. As a keynote speaker, consultant, or in-house trainer, I used to tell my audiences two things:

Firstly, "Fools learn from their own mistakes and wise men learn from others," as my sister is quoted saying. I would let my audience know I was qualified to teach them because I had made every mistake you can make, so they were the wise sitting in front of a fool! (It got a laugh!) In the same vein I share the mistakes we made caring for Mom and Dad and what we learned. And this is my way of teaching you.

Secondly, I couldn't help my chosen career path because growing up my role models were teachers or preachers, so I caught a passion for delivering information in a fast paced, high energy way from my preacher Dad and my teacher Mom. My creative imagination came from my mother's claim that before I was born she prayed for a blue-eyed blond who would love art and music. My mother described me as having a very 'active imagination'.

Growing up in India as Missionary Kids meant that we learned to be innovative and do the best we could with what we had. This went into high gear when I took on the full time responsibility of being their primary caregiver.

I'm the oldest child, the "big bossy sister" with a personality that can be intimidating, but gets the job done. In the native Indian language, I learned as a child, their word for desire is "eetcha". It reminds me of our English word "itch". I often thought of this, especially when I could feel burnout and anxiety threatening my commitment. Deep inside I knew I had to "scratch the itch" because I had this desire or "eetcha" to manage Mom and Dad's care.

Done With Dementia

When they were still living in their own home each of us four kids visited them off and on. My brother Eldon was a Missionary in Bangladesh for fourteen years, returning and living in Calgary in 2004, and my sister Susie and Dr. Terry returned to Canada from the Middle East in 2006. My youngest brother Gary and his wife Janice moved to his in-laws farm just north of Calgary about one hour away. We moved back from Toronto in 2005. So it wasn't until those years that we were able to get a good idea of how Mom and Dad were managing as they aged.

My point is that when Mom and Dad were just surviving day-today with dementia, we didn't know how long they would live, or if they would suffer more physically and mentally. The question was often asked, "What are they living for?" I believe one of the reasons was so we could enjoy being a family, maybe for the first time, with our parents. I felt like God was making up for all the time I lost being with my mother and father as a child in boarding school.

We gathered together and took on the roles and responsibilities of being our parent's main caregivers. We were brought closer to Mom and Dad and to each other. Because our parents saw each of their children at least one weekend a month, they didn't forget who we were. Sometimes our names eluded them, and they got things mixed up, but the joy in their faces and the embrace of their arms said it all.

My mother often said, "You're so beautiful." To which I would reply, "That's because I have a beautiful mother." She'd smile but not take the compliment so I often wondered if she knew it was her I was talking about. She also referred to me as, "My darling!" I used to tell people, "If you were called "my darling" several times every day, you'd take care of them too!" It all made up for boarding school. It also made up for the differences in the cultures we lived in because we became that rare family that chose to look after our parents and keep them in their own home. We did what we wanted to do. Keep them together.

Helping from a Distance

They loved their little house. It was a raised bungalow and they had a mortgage burning ceremony at one of their wedding anniversary celebrations. Their house was on a corner, painted a sunny yellow and Dad had built a double garage facing the alley as the City of Calgary dictated. Neighbors got used to picking raspberries that grew through the fence along the sidewalk. If the neighbors didn't pick berries they were usually gifted with a jar of Mom's homemade jam or jelly. They loved their neighborhood. Mom and Dad were acquainted with them all and happy to participate in the annual street picnic. We could tell story after story of things they did for the neighbors and how the neighbors kept an eye out for them too.

It was a typical two-bedroom, L-shaped living-dining floor plan.

The kitchen had been customized for the former owner, a lady they knew, who had passed away peacefully in the house. When the family was settling her estate and wondering about the house, Dad was just retiring from the ministry and the connection was made. The family made a special deal with Mom and Dad who were delighted to have a home of their own again.

Mom often made the comment, "I'm not moving again! They will have to carry me out of here on a stretcher into a hearse." She did her usual to make the home comfortable, cozy and welcoming for as many family and friends they could cram in as often as possible.

Done With Dementia

Each time I came to visit from Toronto or on my way through for business, I stayed with them. Some of the things in their home needed upgrading or minor renovation. Half the basement was finished with a big bathroom across from a very large room that looked and functioned as a "hotel" room. It had two double beds and a Murphy bed built into a desk unit. Up to six people could sleep there. This was important to Mom and Dad to accommodate our family and the many friends who came through town. All were invited, and sometimes pressured, to stay over.

The unfinished part of the basement was the laundry area and storage. The area Dad used for his clock repair shop and office was on a raised floor for warmth and comfort. Dad spent a lot of time down there working on clocks and watches. When customers came, they went straight down the stairs from the back door, avoiding the rest of the house.

One of my main concerns was that these stairs were very steep and had been carpeted over carpeting. This made the stairs very unsafe especially if you were carrying a laundry basket as Mom had to. She had weak ligaments in her shoulders and could no longer even style her hair, so I wanted to prevent any accidents. I was determined to help in some way even though I was living in Toronto.

It was at this time that I took a closer look at the bathroom upstairs and realized it needed a good update remodel. I also made a note that on the other side of the tub taps and drain was a small closet in the second bedroom. I measured it up and it was just the right size for a stacking washer and dryer. My brother Gary is a Journeyman Electrician and was available to do the hook ups, and my other brother, Eldon, was able to find a stacking unit at the Habitat for Humanity warehouse. This meant that I didn't worry any longer about Mom slipping on the steep steps into the basement with baskets of laundry.

I discovered that CMHC (Canada Mortgage and Housing Corporation) had a program called HASI (Home Adaptations for Seniors' Independence). It gave grants to seniors for home improvements. I checked into this and applied. I spoke with a nice lady who was most anxious to see us get this funding for their bathroom. Imagine our annoyance when Mom and Dad didn't qualify based on their income being too high by $120. Dad just laughed and figured he'd "arrived"! But the bathroom didn't get changed.

I came out for a whole week to do nothing but paint every room of their house in the colors of my mother's choice. I was taping around the doors when Mom came in and asked if she could help do anything. I told her she could help me finish the taping. She hollered down the stairs to Dad, "Johnny! Linda needs help." I immediately told Mom not to bother Dad. He was always so busy and spent every available minute in his clock shop finishing customer's jobs and saving money for as many road trips as possible. Each trip was declared "the last one."

Dad's social inclination meant that on any given day if friends or family weren't stopping by, you'd find the mail lady or the housekeeper, or some other neighbor sitting at the table for a sandwich or a snack. When I was there to paint, Dad invited me to come join them. I said, "Dad, I can't. I'm on a mission." The next day, when one of the guests asked about me joining them, I overheard him say, "She can't. She's on a mission."

While painting the dining room, I noticed that the carpet came half way up the baseboard. I couldn't pull the carpet up because it had been tacked down. I went over to lift a heat vent cover off the floor. Sure enough, there was three quarter inch, solid oak hardwood floors. I began to plan having carpet taken up and the floors refinished.

My husband and I filled half a large coffee can with staples from the underlay of at least two carpet jobs to get it ready for the professionals. We stored all the large pieces of furniture and accessories in the sun porch and kitchen. Mom and Dad went away for three weeks to visit friends and family. The housekeeper was thrilled, declaring they would be healthier and happier in the new environment. Her job would be easier too.

I personally paid for all the things I could afford for these ventures. I knew all the sacrifices my parents had made for me; my education, my music lessons, and other things they did on a regular basis. Dad was always the first to give me a little gift of cash as I stepped into the airport for a trip or took Mom shopping on a girls' day out. He was very generous. He was always picking up the bill before anyone else could. Several of his friends financially better off, complained to me that Dad wouldn't give them a chance to treat because he was always picking up the bill before they could.

It just matched his heart. He followed the principle of sowing and reaping. He also believed that "To whom much has been given, much is required." And he felt he had been given much in life. He always counted his blessings. It was a pleasure for me to give back into his life and look after as much as I could even from a distance.

I was often blessed to have all-expense-paid assignments by clients that took me to or through Calgary. I remember telling Dad this was because I was considered an "expert" in my field of

Merchandising and Display. Dad would humble me and bring me into reality by telling me that an "expert" is a "little spurt that has been!" He was always quick to share a saying or make a comment that would bring truth with humor. No wonder so many people loved my parents as their pastor, friend, or neighbor.

Catching the Clues

Mom's Crisis: I asked my siblings to do video interviews to recall some of their experiences in the caregiving of Mom and Dad. The first question was, "What was the first sign you remember that either of them manifested any symptoms of dementia?" Every single one of them said the time when Mom got lost coming home the few blocks from the grocery store. She didn't know where she was or how to get home. She panicked. She prayed and in her belief the Lord showed her the way home.

We all heard about how she collapsed on the floor in the back entrance and called for Dad who was downstairs in his clock shop with a customer. She never went out alone again. That incident was a wake-up call for the entire family and we began to take more notice of other things as well.

Mom was the bookkeeper and accountant in the family. Dad had the checkbook and one of Mom's biggest complaints was that he neglected to fill in the payee. She had to wait until the statement came in and then by process of elimination and matching up the numbers she would know where the checks had gone. If they hadn't cleared the bank, she didn't have a clue. I now believe he may have been experiencing dementia at that point and forgetting to fill in the checkbook.

Done With Dementia

I was at their house one day when Dad showed me the mail. There were several return-to-sender envelopes that had the pay stub with the check turned backwards so that the company's address wasn't visible through the window of the envelope. Dad also said that some of the checks had been returned in the mail because they were the wrong check to the wrong utility. He didn't come right out and blame Mom.

Dad then asked, would I come each month and look after it for him? I began to get involved in their financial affairs from that time on. I organized files in a file box for each monthly bill and for annual insurance and taxes.

Mom had a medical condition called a bowel prolapse and Dad had been insisting that I look "at your Mommy's bottom." So, one day I asked Mom if I could see what her problem was. I was shocked at the amount of bowel protruding. It often bled because she was not wearing proper underwear; she often just put on a pair of panty hose with no comfortable protection. She had some pads but wasn't remembering to use them. Dad was trying to help her but didn't really know how.

I made an appointment to see the doctor. He was sympathetic to her condition, wrote some prescriptions of soothing creams and suggested that she push it in as often as she could. He rather reluctantly had to admit that patients who were much younger, or who had cancer, got priority for surgery. Mom's condition wasn't life-threatening. He did promise to do his best. I wondered if she would remember to use the cream or push in the prolapse. I also wondered how much Dad was going to be able to help her. Her chair at the table had a pillow and now I realized why it was there.

Linda McKendry

Being the praying family that we are, we asked God to make a way. Our faith paid off. Within two weeks, Mom was called in because there was a short time between two longer surgeries with just enough time to do this little repair. There wasn't even time for a proper pre-op exam. We were elated to know this was going to fix Mom's problem.

I share this because several things came out of this hospital visit. One good, and one really bad. The good one was that in the hospital they were following her GP's prescriptions, which included Aricept. Dad had determined it wasn't working to help Mom mentally, so he had discontinued it for her. She perked up so much from her visit in the hospital that we were happy to have her on it for the right reasons. Her GP had to give her a test, and apparently if you scored too high, or too low, you didn't qualify for it. The doctor also gave us the impression people were trying to get their hands on this drug believing it would do more than doctors claimed for mental degeneration.

We found out from testimonials of nurses what no one was claiming publicly. It was actually helping a lot of their patients. Aricept seemed to stabilize patients with dementia making them "brighter" and more aware of their surroundings and reality. Dad had no explanation for why this had been prescribed but Mom hadn't been taking it. He simply said, "It didn't make any difference." I'm not sure what he was expecting! I took over their medication compliance at this time too.

The bad thing was that no one stayed with Mom in the hospital. It was only a one night stay for the type of surgery she had. I was there in the post-op to give Mom her glasses and her teeth, as the doctor had arranged. She seemed fine and happy to see me.

Done With Dementia

I stayed overnight with Dad, so we could go in the morning and bring Mom home. The hospital called early in the morning to please come right away. We rushed to the hospital to find Mom dressed and standing in the hallway outside her room. When she saw Dad, she ran to him like a crazy person and almost knocked him over. She burst out crying as she clung to him saying, "I couldn't find you!"I was surprised at Dad's reaction. He appeared awkward, kind of embarrassed and was pushing her away, and glancing all around. The nurses came to our rescue and led us into her room.

As an aside, this used to often puzzle me. Most of his parishioners would commend his ability to communicate and comfort them. But when it came to his own family, me included, there were times when we wanted the same treatment and it was as if he was a little shy or reluctant. A lot of professional people are like that. They are different at work with customers, clients, and colleagues, then they are at home or with friends, family, and neighbors.

The nurses told us that Mom had gotten dressed during the night in her street clothes and was walking up and down the halls of the "hotel" looking to see which room her Johnny was in. She wanted to leave that hotel. She didn't like it there. By the time we arrived she had caused too much confusion to have her breakfast and had thrown up after taking her medications on an empty stomach. We had to convince her to get back into the gown, so the doctor could check her over before releasing her. Because she had thrown up, it was decided we had time to take her down to the cafeteria for a quick bite before the doctor came on his rounds.

The surprise was the surgeon's intern who came to examine Mom. She was a beautiful, tall, very dark Ethiopian female doctor. Mom was sitting on the side of the bed, so the doctor turned to get an assistant to help Mom lie down. We all watched as Mom flipped her body onto the bed, legs flying, with obviously no need for any assistance. She always had strong legs.

The doctor said that the surgery was "text book" and that the condition of her tissue and ligaments was that of someone half her age. We credit that with their good living and Mom's attention to healthy eating and exercise.

It was at this point we, as a family, made the decision that Mom would never be left alone again. If there was someone there to keep telling her where her Johnny was, and when he was coming back, she was fine. During the day when Dad was out, Mom didn't seem to be anxious. In the evening, however, when he went to his clock club meetings or out for chaplain visitation and left her, she would be crying when he got home. He began to ask one of us to come over and stay with "your Mommy" and we were always happy to comply. At this point we were only applying this rule to being with Mom when Dad was not there.

Dad's Crisis: Dad loved to have his calendar full. He kept a little black book calendar in his pocket and referred to it often. As a pastor who did the most visits of any other in the entire region, he was always being called on and making appointments to see people. He was very social and used to get a bit upset when Mom wanted to stay home. If he insisted, she would take along a book to read, some knitting, crocheting, or other portable craft project.

Being in the local clock club meant that those regular meetings and events were also plotted in his schedule. Mom's main participation was to help a bit at the clock club trade shows, and make beautiful custom wall art from clock parts that have become collectibles and heirlooms.

He always acted like he knew what he was saying, and they were facts. The first time I knew we had a problem with his memory was when he had the entire household searching for his travel itinerary and e-tickets. He was accusing Mom of putting them somewhere and then not remembering where she put them. She was beside herself with worry and scrambling to look in every place she could think of.

I spied a rather tall pile of books and papers next to Dad's chair. I decided to sit in the chair and go through them one at a time. I found the documents at the bottom of that stack... which relieved Mom and put Dad into utter silence. He didn't say sorry to Mom and acted like it was a joke. That was the first time I had to agree with my sister's observation that, "Dad is mean to Mom."

These aren't easy things to disclose, but for the sake of transparency in discussing the issues of dementia, we tell it like it was. We had such a hard time watching Mom continue to be the loving, caring, and helpful mate to Dad when he didn't seem to respect her. We didn't realize the level of frustration he was experiencing trying to take over the role she had always been so faithful in. He was the first to give her cash for shopping so she could buy something nice for herself. He always made sure she had the nice things she liked and often brought home little gifts of jewelry, rings, and knick-knacks he knew she fancied. He had given up expecting her to drive more, even though she did have her license.

Dad often made up the coffee at night with the timer so there would be fresh coffee in the morning. He liked to take a cup to Mom in bed and announce, with a little British accent, "Doth the Queen want her victuals?" However, the stains and warped wood on the coffee cabinet told the story of a carafe not being placed in the receptacle so that the coffee ran out all over the place.

Driving Dad: Dad was still driving the car, and he was driving Mom to do what she had always done to keep up an independent lifestyle.

One day I smelled something rotten in the kitchen and went to check it out, and found a tuna sandwich in the toaster oven. The bread was all curled up and the tuna was green with a very foul smell. Another day I went into the kitchen to make supper for them and found in the freezer an opened package of raw chicken all dried out from freezer burn and not edible. More and more of these things were putting pressure on Dad and making him difficult for Mom to please.

In my own home, we ate sumptuously every evening. My husband is a premier barbecue man and the budget for steaks, chops, ribs, and other high-quality meats is ample. Many nights I could hardly eat knowing what we were having and how difficult it was getting for my parents to make a decent meal. I couldn't cook for them, serve them, clean up and make it home to do dinner with my husband at his preferred time.

Because Dad was a veteran, he was entitled to a small sum of money each month for hiring a housekeeper, someone to mow the lawn in summer, and shovel sidewalks in winter.

There was also an allowance twice a year for window washing. A nice neighbor lady came by to do light housekeeping bi-weekly and was always convinced to stay for coffee or tea after her work.

Her husband had a hip replacement and the only thing he had to say about it was, "I wished I'd done it sooner." Dad was having hip pain but because of his age the doctor said it would have to break on its own before he would be considered for surgery compared to the housekeeper's husband who was still in the work force. Once again, the system has priorities. Pain relief medication was added to Dad's daily prescriptions.

But another thing that helped his hip was his afternoon routine of having naps, which we always did in India. The saying, "Only mad dogs and Englishmen go out in the noonday sun." or the Mexican "Siesta" made afternoon naps become part of a lifetime habit. Dad would tell people he was off for his "horizontal meditation" or "ceiling inspection". After a crisis I will share in another chapter, he was bedridden for thirty-seven days and this resulted in his hip never hurting again! He also lost thirty-seven pounds, so I believe there was a clear connection there.

Dad shared about the day he rushed home from the store and barely made it to the garage with severe diarrhea. He said Mom didn't know what to do to help him. Looking back, I now wonder if he may have been suffering from food poisoning because of the way they were eating. I also wonder if all his drive to keep everything together and stay independent was causing a lot of stress. Time was telling.

Linda McKendry

Living with One of Us Kids

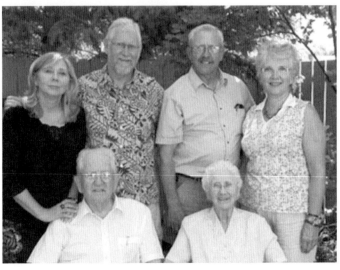

Susie on the far left next to my brother Eldon, then Gary and then me at a relaxed family gathering after the celebrations of Mom and Dad's 60th wedding anniversary, July 2007. Little did we know what kind of a team we would make to care for our parents in this journey.

Each one of us had a different opinion of what kind of care Mom and Dad needed and how to make that happen. We listened to our parents and tried to understand what was important to them and where they needed the most help. The main thing was that they wanted to stay in their own home for as long as possible.

Each of us siblings had spouses and we all had our own families and busy lives. We weren't quite the "sandwich generation" because our children were mostly grown and on their own or in higher education.

Done With Dementia

<u>Jim and I:</u> I am the oldest and my husband and I had moved back from a thirteen year "visit" to Toronto where his corporate transfer had taken him. I took my Visual Merchandising Consulting business with me, built it up in Toronto and brought it back to Alberta. Jim retired after selling his textile converting company.

We live in a very small but well-designed villa home with one bedroom and a den on the main floor and two bedrooms with a bath and large family room in the walk-out basement.

Even though I could imagine fixing up our downstairs space for Mom and Dad to enjoy because they were mobile enough to do the stairs and come up for main meals, my husband was concerned that he would be left to look out for them each day while I was at my office in a commercial district.

He also smoked and even though it wasn't in the house, the cloud of second-hand smoke was never far away. I knew this would be hard for Mom and Dad to endure. I also knew that we couldn't depend on Mom to make snacks or coffee for Dad and they would struggle to feel at home using my kitchen during the day.

I also knew that if I made room for their furnishings and the familiar things they enjoyed, I would have to find a place to store my own. We decided living with us was not a viable option.

<u>Ruth and Eldon:</u> Eldon is a little younger than me. We were the two Mom and Dad had to find care for when they attended the North York Hospital in Toronto to take a course in Tropical Medical Dispensing while getting ready to go to India as Missionaries. Eldon is an aeronautical engineer and natural born mechanic. He and Ruth had spent fourteen years in Bangladesh as missionaries and had recently returned to rent a house they saw

online that turned out to be a lot smaller than it appeared on screen.

They had a house full of young adult children in different stages of school and jobs. They also continued their mission work to a degree and used their home to have meetings and entertain friends and family. The notice from their landlord that he was selling the house coincided with our decision to downsize Mom and Dad and sell their home, which we eventually did. I had contemplated proceeds from the house going to renovate the basement of their home, like what I had envisioned if Mom and Dad lived with us. Ruth and Eldon couldn't see this vision or the prospects of finding a more suitable home for them both to move into. They too, didn't want to move again. The level of care Mom and Dad needed was also a big unknown at that time.

We all knew Dad's intention to give us each some of our inheritance from the proceeds of the sale of their home, so Ruth and Eldon knew they could count on a portion of their down payment from this gift. The timing was tricky, but this motivated them to help with the huge task of downsizing.

Gary and Janice: My brother Gary had retired from a very long career up north in the Oil industry. They had moved onto Janice's childhood farm and into the original farmhouse down the driveway from where her mother and father were living.

Her dad was suffering from extreme symptoms of Parkinson's and Gary and Janice were just a phone call and a few steps from being there to help. He passed away two years after they moved to the farm. This was just at the time when we had the Lodge on the radar of Mom and Dad's next stage of life so offering to take Mom and Dad into their home wasn't even considered.

The other aspect was the distance of the farm from medical services. The original farmhouse was cute and quaint, and Gary and Janice had done a lot of renovations to make it comfortable for the two of them and occasional visits from friends and family. It was not, however, suitable for sharing with Mom and Dad. The main house Janice's mother lived in would have been suitable in terms of space, but that would have been a huge imposition and was not even considered.

Susie and Terry: This is the saddest situation of all. Mom and Dad had traveled back to India and taken Susie and Terry with them. They had a special bond and always talked about having a house or even adjoining units of a townhouse or duplex so Mom and Dad could live close to them.

At the time of our decision making, Susie and Terry, who is a Medical Doctor, were living in a very remote community six hours drive away. While the medical facility there was adequate for average needs, it was an Air Ambulance helicopter ride to the city of Edmonton for a major emergency.

The home provided for them was new and well-appointed. Susie was at home and available for caregiving. Stairs were not a problem for either Mom or Dad to use the bedrooms. The main considerations were all the other services Mom and Dad had and were used to, such as their pharmacist, specialists, hair and foot care professionals. In a place that doesn't even have a decent grocery store, it wasn't wise to make that many changes for people with dementia, who were now in their eighties.

There are also regulations in place that discourage a doctor from treating his own family members. That can be a fine line and if deemed to be crossed could cause Terry to be affected in a negative

Linda McKendry

way. It wasn't worth the risk. Also, because the place is so remote, Susie and Terry headed into the city on days off, and this would mean having to find care for Mom and Dad or take them along.

These were the situations of our current circumstances in terms of offering housing and home care. We proceeded with looking more closely at their own home.

Conditions for Care

It became obvious that while there were some caregiving services in place, like the regular housekeeping, yard care and the snow removal, there were too many things happening daily that were demanding regular or professional oversight.

I called Alberta Health Services (AHS) about Home Care and found out that the levels of care offered were on an hourly basis and included light housekeeping or meal preparation, but no one was available to do both. Also, Mom and Dad were in that place where because they were getting Meals on Wheels and appeared to be so independent it was hard to figure out the exact needs.

Susie, whose husband had served in Abu Dhabi, knew of the Immigrant Social program for Nannies and Nurses. She knew of one woman in particular that she believed we should invite to come and be a live-in nurse. First issue was to look at what accommodations we could offer a live-in nurse. Having a private washroom would be no problem. Once the beds were removed from the "hotel" room with just the Murphy bed and the built-in desk at one end, the room could be refurnished for a private living space.

A kitchenette could be arranged with a bar fridge, a hot plate and a microwave. It was doable, as they say, but not ideal. This would leave the room upstairs where the stacking laundry had been installed for the guest room, or for the nurse to use if she needed to be closer to Mom and Dad for some reason.

The kitchen had been modified by lowering the cabinets to suit the former owner who was in a wheelchair. The layout was not efficient, and the doorways were very narrow. I had measured up the bathroom door when I made the plan for the bathroom upgrade grant and knew that an average size wheelchair would not go through easily. Helping someone bathe would also be challenging.

The house was a raised bungalow and by having a stacking laundry put upstairs in a little closet, there was no need to use the stairs, except for Dad's clock and watch repair workshop. Keeping this in place would be a huge comfort for Dad as there were many pieces, parts, and specialized equipment to sort, or move.

I looked at the space on a regular basis and being in the Interior Design Industry as a Merchandising and Display Consultant

I had some knowledge of how space could be developed and renovated to work better. I saw how a ramp could be built on the outside at the front with access to the parking pad next to the garage for easy mobility if they had to be in wheelchairs.

The big problem was that we needed the equity in their home in order to have the funds to make the house work for them. Both lines of credit and the Home Equity Loan options were available, and the ensuing family discussion was quite animated. There were strong opinions all around.

The big opportunity was that in Calgary the market was at an alltime high with very few properties available for sale and buyers making offers sight unseen. We debated taking advantage of this market condition knowing it would ultimately take a downward turn.

The big statement Dad had made a few years earlier was that when the time came, he would like to live at the Aspen Lodge. As a pastor he would take his turn doing chapel at the Aspen Lodge and several of his fellow parishioners lived there and gave glowing reports about how much they loved it.

The big plan was to begin to downsize them, prepare them for the inevitable move, and list the house if and when that decision needed to be made. We decided it wouldn't hurt to begin to sort and get rid of unneeded items. This is when Dad decided we needed a family meeting to read the will and find out what items we were inheriting so we could take them right away. I believe he thought it was one way to make sure none of the family heirlooms would go missing in the shuffle.

The Family Meetings

At this family meeting, Dad had gotten out their will and a list of every item each of us was to inherit. He had begun to either put a piece of tape, a sticky-note, or a colored dot on the backs or bottoms of things that had one of our names on it. We each had different ideas about this too.

Susie didn't want to think about them dying at all, so she opted out at first, but as Dad began the list and things especially for her were described, she warmed to the purpose of the meeting. Eldon had asked for Dad's pastoral resource and reference library and put dibs on some of Dad's tools, being the mechanical one in the family.

Gary, as I recall, had his eye on a very unusual square shaped porcelain pitcher that had a handle on one of the corners. He asked if he could have it. Later after research he found out it was a very rare memento to Teddy Roosevelt and delighted in telling us what it was worth on eBay. He also did the research about the merchant ship Dad had sailed to India on during the war. He then gave a framed picture to Dad which was returned to him after Dad died.

I began to put my name on a few things here and there that I fancied which mostly fit into my own home décor. Dad began to just give us something to take if we fancied it, or got us to put a sticker on it with our name.

Originally, I had been shy about asking. Then I remembered when my husband's grandmother offered me a huge cast iron skillet. I mean, it was larger than any I had ever seen. I declined, not wanting to appear too eager to take anything from a senior living in a single room Assisted Living Facility. She passed away the following week and of course the skillet was dealt with by a surviving family member and I felt bad that I hadn't taken it when she offered. I know my husband would have enjoyed using it at his hunting camp.

On this occasion, Dad read the list and when he got to one item, he said, "Well, it's got a chip in it, but it's the real thing." Then he came to another item for someone else and it was an old antique chair, "It needs a little repair." And for me, he pointed to an electric clock with an old world motif that had been in my Grandma Thiessen's kitchen on the farm. It was one of the few things my mother had inherited. It had a crack right down the middle that had been glued. But it worked!

Finally, he named an item for Gary and we sat waiting to see what was wrong with it. Nothing. Gary said, "Hey, I feel cheated! Everyone else got something that needs fixing except me!" We all laughed, and it took some of the edge off such a serious discussion.

This was also the night that I spearheaded the discussion on the need for someone to be appointed Enduring Power of Attorney. After I explained it all, they all looked at me as if to say, "So?" And while it felt scary, I offered, on the condition that another one of us would be a backup. Eldon, who also lived in Calgary, accepted, and that arrangement gave me more confidence to take on the main role and responsibility.

I arranged to sign them up immediately, knowing that we needed to put these things in place while they were of reasonable mental clarity. I took over more and more responsibility for things as required, including arranging a tour for all of us of the Aspen Lodge, downsizing, listing the house, and eventually moving them.

I appreciated that at each family meeting we were forthright and honest in giving our opinions and looking for solutions that would work for Mom and Dad with the least amount of upset in our individual lifestyles. Dad always expressed his desire to make sure that whenever he benefited financially, he wanted each of his children to have a portion.

When the downsizing made the house look too empty and vacant, there was a sudden panic on Dad's part. We called another meeting to talk about it. He nodded in understanding when we explained the situation with Ruth and Eldon and their need for the down payment from the sale of the home. He didn't say anything after that, but you could see the conflict as Dad wanted to help

Ruth and Eldon, but he also didn't seem ready to move. I felt like he wanted everything to slow down a little and looking back I recall what a hard decision it was.

We didn't know about all the home care that was ultimately available to us, which might have made a difference. My active mind could imagine using funds from the sale of the house to renovate Ruth and Eldon's house to accommodate Mom and Dad but they weren't buying into it.

Besides, Mom and Dad's names were on the waiting list at the Lodge with two opportunities to refuse until their names would go to the bottom of the list again. It was all so overwhelming at the time and the easiest decision seemed to be moving forward so Mom and Dad could get into the Lodge.

Susie recalls that we had promised Mom and Dad that we wouldn't put their house up for sale and they could move back into it, if their lifestyle in the Lodge wasn't working. That was before Ruth and Eldon's landlord announced that he was putting up their house for sale. Among all the pros and cons was the fact that the market was so strong for selling and would give Mom and Dad the maximum return on their investment. I also knew it would give us more resources for whatever we would need and that was a comfort all around.

It was a tough meeting. On one hand Dad wanted Ruth and Eldon to be able to purchase the home they were in. On the other hand, he was disappointed that they didn't want to make arrangements for him and Mom to come and live with them. He was facing moving to the Lodge, which he knew had been his suggestion, and we didn't know if we had gone too far down the downsizing road to turn back.

There were still dishes in the kitchen and pots and pans under the stove. Their bedroom was all intact except for the clothes already hanging in the portable wardrobes. They were still having light meals and daily naps in the house, but just to look around anyone could see that the house wasn't looking like the home they had for so many years.

We also saw Mom's inability to make decisions or even understand what was happening. She realized she suffered dementia more than Dad. We kept telling her again and again what was happening and since she took all her cues from Dad, the bottom line was that wherever her Johnny was going, she was going with him. That was all that mattered to her.

It was the way they depended on each other over the years that so heavily influenced our decisions. Most big decisions Mom left up to Dad and just followed and supported him. Dad, however, depended on Mom for a lot of daily things and if we were there pitching in for what she would have been looking after he didn't complain or put any pressure on her. If she wasn't doing anything, he would often say, "Lydia, get helping!" And she would jump up quick to go in the direction he was pointing, but not sure exactly what she was supposed to do when she got there.

She would come over to where we were sorting things, often handling and touching trinkets on a table next to a pile of packing paper and make comments as though she was browsing at a flea market. Most of the time she didn't express any ownership or memories of the items. She even said once, "I wonder where this came from." We would struggle to remember if it had some story or person behind the gift or purchase so we could help her remember. Many things we didn't have a clue. One pat answer she always accepted was, "Dad probably picked it up at a garage sale."

And she would nod and smile, accepting that explanation if we said so.

Susie recalls trying to sort books so Mom could take her favorites or ones she hadn't read yet to the Lodge and the rest would go into the donate pile. She would look over at Mom reading the first page, over and over, before she realized that Mom might never read an entire book again. It was a sad time, but also a revealing one.

For Dad, as a minister who had a whole library full of reference books and Bible commentaries, it was easier. Eldon was to get them all. He had the legacy of the father's business so that was a given. I'm also a collector of books and several times when I visited from Toronto, Dad would point to a suitcase full of books and ask me to go through them and take what I wanted because the rest were going to the Good Will. I would start to sort and then decide I wanted them all. After all, how can you tell if you want a book or not if you haven't read it? Some of them are still in my library today. Some are very old, dating back to the late 1800's, and many have inscriptions in the fly leaf with names and dates of the givers and the receivers. Some of the names I recognize and many I don't, but the stories are priceless and take me back to my childhood and even to my parent's world as children, and I value the history.

This really motivated me to make sure that their new home was as cozy, comfortable, and as functional as possible. I took great pains to make sure everything was measured up, that it fit on the plan, and they would feel as much as possible like they were home. They each had their own chairs. Dad's recliner had an electrical device to help push the seat up so it was easier to get in and out of.

Linda McKendry

He really loved his chair. Mom's matched it in color and style but was smaller.

Their chairs faced the entertainment center with the TV, lots of ornaments, framed family pictures, some books, and the bottom shelf from end-to-end with photo albums Mom had done over the years. Adjacent was the wall with the bay window and at the Lodge I made sure this was the identical arrangement only the adjacent wall with the window was on the other side. The cable outlet in the suite dictated where to place the furniture.

Without the funds from the house, we couldn't afford the care or any modifications to make the house better for what they needed. Without the funds, Ruth and Eldon couldn't make a down payment on the house they didn't want to move out of or modify. Without the funds I wasn't free to make decisions for them that involved finances for more than basic rent and utilities that could be covered by their pensions.

We assumed that moving into Assisted Living provided a safe place to live that supplied meals and light housekeeping. They would have enough independence and ability to do the things they really enjoyed, like trips to visit friends and family, church and brunch on Sundays. This would be necessary so they could avoid bingo, dancing, bridge, and other typical senior activities they were not familiar with or comfortable participating in.

Counting the Cash

Finances always play a major role in decision making at all stages of life. Those with great faith learn to trust God and move forward where they feel led. My parents were in that category. In India, as missionaries in the rural West Bengal state about 200 miles from

78

Calcutta (Kolkata), we learned as adults that they had lived on our school allowance and sent us to boarding school on their salary.

We were the poorest kids in the school with the least number of extras beyond the required clothes, shoes, and school supplies. This was verified at one of my class reunions in the U.S. The Gambles were known to be the least affluent and from the denomination that supported their missionaries the least. Our parents were givers. They believed in tithing, which is giving back to God 10% of their income, and this they did religiously.

Dad had spent time in the Merchant Marines which is when he felt the Divine calling on him to go back to India where they had docked on a military mission during the war. He signed up to be a Marine Engineer, which ultimately meant that you shoveled coal on the ship in the engine room on shifts. Dad was so unlike other typical sailors and not anxious to go to shore for the "wine, women, and song" that he was often chosen by the ship's captain to stay aboard and mind the ship when it was in dock.

You can imagine his surprise and joy when the Canadian Government finally recognized the Merchant Marines as veterans deserving of pensions and pay when he received a large check in the mail for back pay. He immediately re-roofed the house and gave each of us kids $1,000. It was also at that point that the Veterans Aid kicked in to provide him an ongoing allowance for housekeeping, summer and winter yard maintenance, hearing aids and eye glass prescriptions. Later on, medical and sanitary supplies were also covered, saving us hundreds of dollars each month.

Along with the cash he collected from his clock and watchmaking and repair business, he was flourishing and putting away enough for him and Mom to take many "last trips" on the road to visit friends and relatives. The pension he got from the church when he retired was not enough to support him into the later years, but they did have an investment program with interest rates higher than the banks at that time and he invested in that. He was also an agent for an insurance company and had a few contracts from which he got annual returns. They weren't lacking and were able to pay off their mortgage.

The first time I sat down with Dad to collect all the bank statements and other "chits" to take to the friend who did their income tax returns, I was shocked at how much they gave to registered charities, friends, and family, in addition to the ten percent tithe to their local church. I remarked about it to Mom and she said, "Oh yes. That's what Dad does. The harder things get, the more he gives away." I totaled the receipts I had for donations to be used for income tax: it was just over 20% of his income for that year.

He would never think of visiting someone, on church duty or personally, without taking something, especially if he was visiting unannounced. It was usually something good to eat with the expected tea or coffee offer. And he wasn't shy to always offer to pay for everyone's meals. For one of their anniversaries, he took the entire family to the town where he had first pastored, where he had met my mother, and where they were married. He paid for the old-fashioned steam train ride that they conduct there for tourists each summer and a sumptuous meal after with a little program in the local community center.

In addition to giving and entertaining as much as possible in their own home, he also was a good receiver. People would come by and bless them regularly with gifts, food, and watches to either repair or fix to sell. Many times friends would invite them to concerts, plays, and other events and pay their way. As a retired itinerate preacher, he was also asked to fill the pulpits of ministers who were on holidays, sabbatical, or ill and he always received generous honorariums for that.

He was extremely generous with Mom. He made sure she always had cash in her purse for shopping and they had credit cards to use for travel and vehicle expenses. Dad had a saying he got from his mother, "There are only three things to avoid in life... Debt, Dirt, and the Devil," so he avoided debt and always paid his credit card statement at the end of each month. Or I should say got Mom to do it, since she kept the books and paid the bills.

Mom had her own honorariums from speaking engagements for women's groups, and at one time when they were pastoring a church that had split and couldn't afford the pastor, she worked at a local variety store in a small community. It was at that time that Dad was voted on the local hospital board, which paid for the meetings and travel expenses when required. Mom was invited to teach a course on Christianity for religious studies at the local High School and was paid for doing that as well. They were industrious and had a good work ethic.

Even though Mom never made money selling what she made, she was a master at saving money. Her jams and jellies were coveted as gifts. Her knitted sweaters were appreciated and enjoyed by all who got one and she did a lot of sewing and made home décor items instead of buying them readymade. She could make meals go a long way and was always baking something to serve for the almost daily times Dad invited someone home without telling her first.

Linda McKendry

So even though they weren't rich by any means, they were frugal and generous, and seemed to have everything they needed and wanted. Dad had another saying, "Do your giving while you're living, so you're knowing where it's going." His idea, which he expressed quite freely was that the day he died he would have spent his last cent, but he also wanted to make sure his children benefited from all he could do while he was still alive.

I was operating my consulting business and traveling a lot at that time with a contract I had with a textile supplier to train decorators of a Canadian chain department store. As I traveled, and as fate would have it, I kept sitting by people who were parenting their parents. I remember the gist of the conversations began to have a common thread through them. One was to live as close to them as possible and care for them yourself if you could. The second was to let them give away as much as they could to their heirs while they had it, or to have joint accounts with their heirs, so the government couldn't take it all to care for them, leaving nothing for the children.

I kept hearing stories about how many parents' nest eggs were dwindled down because of health care and living costs and the parents didn't have any to leave to their children. The other dichotomy was that some of the best care went to the people who could least afford it compared to compromised care for those who could afford expensive, high end facilities. This was confusing to me. I knew that in Canada we have automatic Old Age Pensions and Canada Pension Plans for people who had paid into the plan when they were in the workforce.

It began to look like there was a need to balance the amount of money on hand with what someone could risk giving away to the heirs while they were still alive. We had made the arrangements for the Aspen Lodge care based on line 250 of their income tax returns before they sold the house, so they qualified for financial assistance and the cost for the two of them was very reasonable and affordable. We knew that with the sale of the house, it wouldn't be an issue.

I asked the question, "Does it matter what they get for the sale of their home?" I was told, "No. The only thing that matters is what is on line 250 of their income tax return year to year." Based on that, Dad took 50% of the revenue from the sale of the house, divided it in four and gave each of us kids our "inheritance," saying he didn't know how long he would live and that might be all we were getting. The other half I invested in a church fund that was still earning more interest than the banks at that time.

The way it worked out, the income on line 250 on their tax return was only calculating income from the interest on the funds from the house and what Dad had put in there all along, combined with their Canada Pensions and Old Age Security, so they were usually well within the combined income for a couple to qualify for the subsidies and programs.

This turned out to be such a blessing. After we moved them out of the Lodge, I felt all the pressure of managing their finances. My brother Gary and I came up with a plan that assumed they would live to one hundred at the expenses we had caring for them in their own home. We calculated what we needed above and beyond the Canada Pension and Old Age Security. We added some of the Self Managed Care funding we had coming in for the nurse. We then figured out the difference between that and the monthly expenses for their rent, utilities, groceries, and miscellaneous and asked for that amount from the fund for six months at a time... bi-annually.

Linda McKendry

We asked the agent to make it automatic, which he did. This plan worked for us to the end of their lives.

After their estate was taken care of by the executor there were sufficient funds for each of us to have just over $10,000 each. I could see Dad smiling from heaven, happy that he hadn't gone to his death penniless, in poverty, or without anything to leave to his children and his children's children.

We promised Mom and Dad that after six months at the Aspen Lodge, if they weren't happy and it wasn't working out, we would move them into their own home again. We knew that with the available funds from the house and what they had put away, we could make some arrangements for them.

THE MOVING PLAN

Sorting the Stuff

When I recall all the stuff we had to sort and dispose of it reminds me of what their lifestyle was like. Mom had special places for organizing her sewing, needle crafts, letter writing, card sending, gift wrapping, and equipment for all the jams and jellies she made on a regular basis. From that point of view, she had so many things already "sorted," which made it easier to make decisions on her behalf considering her level of dementia even then.

We made sorting and packing an almost full-time job in those days. I had measured up their space at the Aspen Lodge and had figured out what furnishings to move to make their new place as similar to what they were used to. We had three piles: one to keep, one to give away, and one to sell. At least that was our plan. We all pitched in even though there were differing opinions of what was worth keeping, selling, or donating to goodwill.

Done With Dementia

Mom's dementia was advanced enough that she didn't have her usual hospitality hat on, which meant she wasn't concerned about making coffee or lunch as we worked. Dad would come in from time to time and say, "Lydia, make us some coffee. Are there any biscuits?" Mom would startle, look a little confused, and head for the kitchen with one of us following her to make it happen. We didn't want Dad getting cross at her. Besides those little interruptions she pretty much kept doing the same thing.

She would pick up a book or an ornament and make a comment that revealed she didn't have any special memory about it. We knew differently about some things, so that was proof to us about her memory. However, when she had a story to tell or a comment about specific items, it would remind us that she was still fond of some things and they had relevant meaning to her in the moment. Because we knew that "out of sight would definitely be out of mind" we still placed some of these things in the donate pile.

Take the laptop, for example. I recall when Dad purchased a laptop for Mom to use instead of her word processor that had replaced her old typewriter. The ink-tape cassettes for use in the word processor were no longer available. She was so frustrated about this change and huge learning curve. Several times Dad asked me to come over and "show your Mommy" how to use the computer. I think that if it had been a desktop with a more normal keyboard, that might have been easier for her, but she never did get the hang of it and just quit writing. Dad took up trying to type his Bible study notes on the laptop and was getting quite skilled at it. Everything we touched brought back a memory and confirmed why things were changing. I decided to put the laptop in the "keep" pile.

Linda McKendry

My sister and I have vastly different opinions of what is "trash" and what is "treasure" to be salvaged. Maybe I've had to do more with less over the years than she has. Her turn at helping Mom and Dad resulted in several large black garbage bags she designated for the trash. I took one look in them and immediately put them over into the "donate" pile!

We tried to have Mom and Dad available for all this sorting so they could help make decisions. Dad was trying to get into the swing of things by sorting through all his clock and watchmaker's tools, and some old papers and documents.

Packing Is a Process: Packing is not an easy job. My mother was a master packer. When I was growing up, I watched her and then helped her make the lists of everything she packed in the trunks and barrels that were shipped to India. She was so clever to nest things or take items out of their store packaging to make more room. I remembered her cutting out brand names or instructions from packaging and tucking them in with items for reference later.

Jim and I had corporate moves where the moving company brought their people in with packing, boxes, labels, and everything needed to pack up an entire household and move to another city. I decided to knock down all the boxes and crates and store them in case we ever needed them. I also decided to flat fold each piece of packing paper and store that also. That included the bright pink tissue paper used to identify something really small or delicate to keep it from accidently getting thrown out.

Within weeks of our stuff arriving in Mississauga, Ontario in our new home, Mom and Dad came out for a visit. Naturally Dad asked if he could help. I showed him the stack of packing paper piled to the ceiling in our large unfurnished dining room and said,

"I want all that flattened, smoothed out, folded and stacked to store." He promptly got two TV trays, two chairs and set up in a corner to begin the task. Of course, he wrangled Mom into the task, but it was so cute to walk by and see both of them in there chatting and laughing as they arranged the monstrous pile of packing paper.

For our move back to Alberta from Ontario I did such a good job of packing that the movers said they were amazed at how balanced and easy the boxes were to carry. I give all the credit to my mother and have been able to help other friends and family with these tricks. Having such a good supply of boxes and packing paper made the process a whole lot easier.

The Waiting List

Qualifying for Assisted Living:

The process of considering the Aspen Lodge for Mom and Dad's new lifestyle involved taking a tour of the facilities, getting all the information including the costs, and having an interview.

The Aspen Lodge is a beautiful, well-designed and well appointed facility in the care level called Assisted Living for Seniors. It's like living in a grand hotel, with high vaulted ceilings over a central common area just off the main entrance. The amenities include a chapel, exercise rooms, a small tuck shop, and even a hair salon/barbershop. There are lots of notices of planned programs and activities. The grounds have manicured lawns, beautiful mature trees, safe sidewalks, and good parking for staff, residents, and visitors.

Instead of typical hotel rooms there are one room studio suites. These are without kitchens where a single senior can live with all their down-sized personal belongings and mementoes. Every other unit has a walk-in shower alternating with a unit that has a tub. If you are a single senior, they try to give you your preference of tub or shower. Of course, in each room there is also an emergency pull cord for immediate assistance. For couples, two rooms are joined by an unlocked doorway between them. Some couples each have a room as a bed-sitting room and spend most of their day at one of many special activity rooms or alcoves; reading in front of a fireplace, playing games, doing puzzles, or even baking cookies in a kitchen dining area on one of the floors.

Weekly light housekeeping is included and this was to be scheduled on the day the residents signed up for the laundry room. The idea is that while you are doing your laundry, your room is being dusted and vacuumed. The rule was that all the personal items on top of surfaces have to be temporarily moved for the dusting to be done, and that includes the window ledges. Most residents just pile these items on their beds or chairs. Waste baskets are to be emptied by residents and they are shown the garbage chute by the storage units on each floor. There are also rules as to what kind of items cannot be disposed of for various health and safety reasons.

The main consideration for us was the daily meal service. The Lodge provided three meals a day and three snacks. The number of residents dictated that there were two sittings in the dining room for meals and, except for breakfast, the times were scheduled and the seating assigned. It was buffet style and if a resident wasn't mobile enough for the self-serve, a staff member was available to assist.

The first qualification for Mom and Dad was their age and stage in life relative to their state of health and mobility. They were also applying as a couple. This meant that a vacancy of two adjoining suites would have to be available. There was a very small percentage of couples and when either spouse passed away or had to be moved into a higher care facility, the one left would be moved to a single unit, so the adjoining units could be rented for couples.

Each room had its own locked door so in the case of couples they had a "back door" and a "front door" of sorts. We planned for Mom and Dad to set up one unit as a living area and the other as the sleeping one. The bathroom off the living area was used for guests and the one off the bedroom for their private use. This meant there were also two closets, two windows to the outside and extra storage space for off season clothes, suitcases, and stuff not used every day.

The units were unfurnished. So it was up to us to help Mom and Dad decide how to furnish their space. This included wall décor, photo albums, DVDs and videos and other little things like bedside clocks, lamps, games, and books. I decided to include a little cabinet for a coffee station and a place to keep their meds beside a little drop leaf table with two chairs for them and two folding chairs for company. It all seemed to make sense and when I showed my plan to Dad he nodded in apparent understanding and approval. Mom just said, "That's interesting, dear," as if I was showing her a client's project.

The second qualification that I worried about the most was the actual cost. As it turned out, based on Line 250 of their joint tax return, they qualified for "assistance" and the cost was affordable. Access to all the amenities was free, even though some had to be signed up for. The hair salon operated like any other. The parking space, phone, and cable was extra, but two of those three Mom and Dad had been paying for anyhow.

Their pensions alone would cover the basic cost and once the house sold, they would have ample funds to cover other costs. Dad's decision to pay off the car loan was at the top of the list, after giving each of us kids part of our inheritance. They didn't have a mortgage on their home and other funds invested, so financially I felt confident this would be an affordable move. They were still somewhat independent, taking drives and little trips to visit out of town friends and family. Dad used the credit card mostly for gas in the car and some expenses for his watch repair business.

The third qualification was an interview before they would be put on the waiting list. We were told that a three to six month waiting for couples was average.

With the symptoms of Mom's dementia and Dad's issues with Mom, I was concerned how the interview would go. I wasn't worried, being their EPOA. I assumed I would be included in the interview. I was wrong. They interviewed Mom and Dad alone and it was one hour long.

I waited anxiously with thoughts of other places we could explore as options, not knowing if or when their house would sell. When the interview was over the Manager came out smiling, shook my hand, and told me they came through with flying colors and arranged for me to come into her office and sign the documents with them.

Later I asked Dad what kind of questions they had asked him. "The usual", was his reply. I said, "Like what?" "Oh, to make sure we would get along with the other residents!" I left it at that, because Mom and Dad's social habits were the least of my concerns. Apparently, the Manager explained the rules and what they would be allowed to do or not do and I guess she believed that Mom and Dad understood it all. I knew Dad would be nodding and Mom would be going along with Dad, smiling a lot and appearing to be engaging, no matter what.

We were given a list of all the services that could be hired privately, which included laundry, medication reminders, and outings if you didn't use your own transportation. As a family, we believed they would take advantage of the amenities and enjoy the overall ambiance of the Lodge. I imagined them using the exercise rooms, spa, library, games room, and lounge with a fireplace and a little common room with a kitchen and beverage dispenser for coffee, tea, hot water, or hot chocolate 24/7. I imagined that this would be perfect for when they had visitors, which was the norm for them.

They were happy to give away pieces of furniture to family members who were delighted to receive them. The beautiful buffet and hutch were given to one of my cousins who was a Mary Kay director. She was able to use it to showcase and store her beauty products in her suite, so it found a perfect home.

Linda McKendry

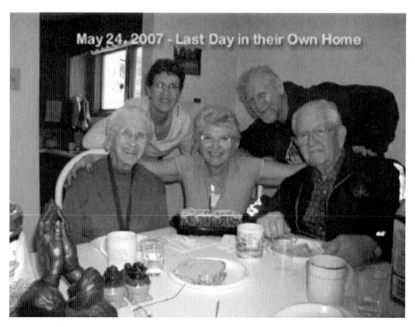

May 24, 2007 - Last Day in their Own Home

Now it was just a matter of time for their names to come up as we kept sorting and downsizing while sourcing a good mover. Each evening when I left them in their ever-emptying house, I wondered how they were feeling, but I was glad we had a plan. Being proactive and ready for any crisis brought me a lot of peace of mind.

LIFE IN THE LODGE

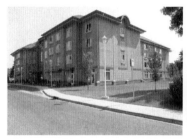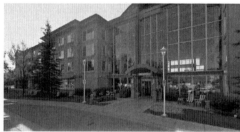

Paradise is Not Perfect

We moved them in the end of May. It coincided with the closing of the sale of their home within days of each other. For the first month they were getting settled and I was going over as often as I could and calling often. Dad always answered the phone, leading me to believe that everything was fine. In July we celebrated their 60th wedding anniversary and made it special by renting an old Vintage Car. All the residents at the Lodge were at the main entrance to see the car pull up and see them dressed up. I got an old-fashioned bowler hat for dad and a rimmed lacy hat for mom with ribbon tied under her chin. The reception and program was in the hall attached to their home church which was only a few blocks away. Later we met as a family at Ruth and Eldon's for a quiet backyard visit, to go through the hundreds of greeting cards, and enjoy some of the leftover food. Dad drove Mom back to the Lodge in their own car. It all seemed all right.

Linda McKendry

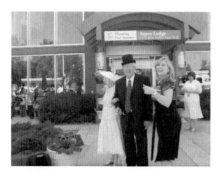 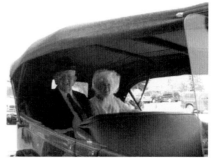

When we were going through the Lodge on the tour, everything looked perfect. In addition to all the amenities, services, and beautiful surroundings, we encountered many residents in various activities who looked happy and contented. Each time we took a different floor to see something else offered, we would see at least one person sitting at a table working on one of the many puzzles laid out for fun.

Most of the residents were navigating with their walkers or canes and several had motorized scooters. Everything seemed to be what any elderly couple would enjoy. They had traveled the world and rarely stayed in places as nice as this and this was where they would actually be living. There is a saying, "How you do anything, is how you do everything!" The place seemed ideal.

Many times, while I was on the phone with him, or even visiting in person, the intercom system in each room would announce an event or reminder. We had been told it was there so that emergency instructions would be clearly heard. This turned out to be an annoyance for Dad especially when it disturbed his afternoon naps. It would also scare Mom when Dad wasn't there to explain what was happening.

Done With Dementia

What had given me so much comfort knowing that help would be close by, was turning into a major annoyance for both. It also made me wonder if the staff could listen in on the residents.

I had purchased a portable keyboard and stand along with earphones so Mom could still enjoy playing the piano without disturbing any of the adjoining residents. Mom couldn't remember how to turn it on and mostly wanted to play it when Dad wasn't there for something to do. She had long stopped playing her favorite videos because she couldn't remember how to get the equipment working. She was more and more dependent on Dad for their entertainment or TV watching. Also, the TV cable they now had was a different supplier than what they had at their own house, so even the news was on a different channel.

Each time I came by, it was easier to just trot down to the end of the hall and make coffee, tea, or hot chocolate from the machine in the kitchen, especially with the free and fresh creamers in the fridge. We could either sit at one of the tables and enjoy the second floor view, or take beverages back to their room. Each time their doors would close, they would automatically lock and I'd have to knock or take one of their keys to get back in. It reminded me of a hotel in that regard.

We were told when we did the tour that there were residents who used the community kitchen in the morning to have the breakfasts they were used to, like making their own porridge or eating at a certain time. We thought this would work for Dad because they were only a few doors down from the community kitchen. Dad had been making their favorite breakfast oatmeal, adding flax seeds, raisins, or dates, milk and brown sugar, when they still lived at home. Whether he never realized he could do this at the Lodge, or just didn't want to, we never found out. It's hard to change your ways and having someone else cook for you makes it easier to take advantage of that.

They were usually sitting in their chairs and watching their favorite DVDs or movies. I would look at the big calendar on the wall and see what events and activities were coming up for the month. I would ask them which ones they were planning on participating in and I began to make plans to be there for some of them. Since evenings were easier for me to get up to the Lodge. I was often heading down to the common room for the 8:00 pm snack time of coffee and cookies. As the residents sat around the scattered tables, staff would come by with a coffee cart to offer tea or coffee with the condiments and an assortment of home-made baked goods fresh each day from the main kitchen.

Meals could be arranged to be eaten with family or guests and they had separate seating depending on the number of people being served. Even though they would try and accommodate "walk-ins," they preferred that you registered your guests for meals ahead of time. There was a nominal cost for these meals, which was under $10. Snacks were free for guests.

The two things I noted were the quality and nutritional value of the food. As a typical buffet there was always soup and salads along with a main entre of meat and vegetables and desserts. I watched as the residents filed through the line and noticed that many of the more mobile ones were just taking one course at a time back to their assigned seats. Others were using their walkers to set their plates on as they gathered as much as they could in one trip. A few were bent over the tables, wearing bibs, and being helped, or fed by a staff member. This was an indication to me of the level of advanced care available at this facility based on physical disability.

Mom and Dad seemed happy with the menus in the beginning. Then Dad began to mention that he was craving beef that wasn't hamburger. They were also driving over to their favorite East Indian restaurant for a good feed of rice and curry which Mom used to make at least once a week. The few times I ate with them I took note of the type of greens in salads, and other options based on my own health conscious preferences and realized that for Mom and Dad, those things were not significant.

Things that began to happen through August, September, and November are discussed in the next chapters. I don't recall the exact dates of each time a red flag came up, except to say that each time I made note of something, it was just taken care of in the most suitable manner available. Based on "logical" and "loving" things to do, I was still doing my best, while keeping an eye on as much as possible. Without realizing it, we had put even more pressure on Dad to look after Mom and that began to unravel too.

Coffee Pots and Candles

Dad used to call all the walkers "chariots" and chuckle about them getting all lined up just before the meals were served. He was a bit of a flirt and a ladies' man, so he was always ready to entertain the ladies as he walked past them. We never did figure out how Mom felt about it all. She seemed to take all his jokes and antics in stride and still laughed at them until her dying day.

The one thing no resident could have was candles in their rooms. They could have battery operated ones, but nothing with an open flame. This was understandable. However, they were allowed to have a coffee pot in their rooms, or an electric tea kettle. I don't think the little coffee station I set up on the corner of a small hutch we had brought from their house was ever used.

Linda McKendry

One funny story is about waiting for Mom and Dad to come down to the main entrance so we could go out. I sat on a bench between two of the residents and one of them leaned over and said: "We really like it here, but we miss being in the kitchen. I wish they would let us do the dishes occasionally, or even mop a floor!" The lady on the other side leaned really close to me and said in a whisper, "I can show you how to make macaroni and cheese in a coffee maker!" as she nodded seriously. I asked her why she would do that. She said, "Well, you know how we are not allowed to have a hot plate or microwave in our rooms. I love macaroni and cheese, so I figured out how to make it in my coffee maker." It reminded me of the ad showing two guys cooking macaroni and cheese on a car engine!

I remember laughing and thinking how desperate some of these women must be if they missed making macaroni and cheese that badly when beautiful full course meals were made for them three times a day. I also wondered why they wouldn't go use the community kitchen when it had a stove and everything they needed, except the ingredients. More and more things were pointing to the fact that some of the amenities designed into the facility were there more for the family and guests than the residents.

Everything had sounded and looked so nice when we went through our tour and talked with the manager after their interview. The little details caused mostly by dementia, were showing up week after week, and had not been considered problems. We picked Wednesday for their cleaning and laundry day. I wrote it down on the community wall calendar each resident had in their rooms.

Done With Dementia

Aspen Lodge was called "assisted living" because it was a lowlevel care facility. Mom, other than getting up, using the washroom, getting dressed and making the bed, didn't have any awareness of what they would do next. While other residents were busy moving about the halls and participating in spontaneous and planned activities, Mom was just following Dad's lead every minute of the day.

She could not be left alone even then, but we didn't know how severe her dementia was.

Dad was getting more and more impatient with her clinging neediness. While his male ego loved that she adored him and would do everything he said to please him, it was wearing him down having to look after both of them all the time. Other residents began to tell me that they often found Mom sitting on a chair next to the elevator crying and asking everyone who came by, "Have you seen my Johnny?" It turned out that Dad would try to send her up to their room and she didn't have a clue how to get there.

Mom also had trouble getting the laundry done each week on their designated day. She didn't know where to go, what to do, or how to get back to the room. We suspect Dad was trying to help, in his rather gruff way with her, when he got frustrated, and it didn't seem to be making any difference.

There was the time when he called and asked me if I would do the laundry, especially his shirts and underwear. Mom was already wearing pull ups because of her bowel condition so she didn't have as much underwear as Dad. He said he could pay me, and could I come on Wednesday evening too and stay with Mom while he went to clock club? We all knew how important clock club was to Dad, so I made the arrangements even though they were about half an hour away from my home at that time. I didn't promise him he would get his laundry back the same day.

I met my sister-in-law, Ruth, in the hallway as I was coming in on the first Wednesday. "Oh!" I said, "I didn't know you were coming by this evening. Dad asked me to come by and stay with Mom and then asked me if I would take their laundry home and do it. He offered to pay me to do that." She stopped and said, "That's why I'm here too! He called me for the same thing." We laughed and carried on, both of us staying for the evening and playing dominoes with Mom but it showed us clearly that Dad didn't remember that he had already called one of us. Ruth lived closer, so we made arrangements for Wednesday help between the two of us. Dad looked surprised when he came home and apologized, but they were also delighted that we were both there. More for Mom!

I wasn't surprised at this turn of events. On one occasion I came by for a quick call and passed the laundry room where Mom was ironing one of Dad's shirts. She was complaining that it wasn't a very good iron since it wasn't getting the wrinkles out. I looked and it wasn't turned on. I turned it on and went on down the hall to their suite to see Dad for a minute. I had to go to the bank. I stopped again in the laundry room and told Mom I'd be back.

When I came back, there she was still ironing the same shirt, at the same place, and the iron had shut itself off again. I knew that doing laundry for her was a thing of the past. It was confirming that we had to make some changes in that department. Between Ruth and I we covered the laundry, enjoyed the little financial benefit, and kept Dad happy and Mom in peace.

Done With Dementia

They had been to my office many times in the commercial district, especially when Dad would drop Mom off so he could go and do some shopping or visit his clock club buddies. It was on one of those visits I caught another clue that was leading to the truth about the level of dementia in both of them. The most recent day Dad dropped Mom off she was wearing sandals, no stockings, and only had a lightweight sweater. It was during a spring thaw. There was melting snow and puddles in the parking lot.

Knowing that Mom wasn't making good self-care decisions I chided Dad for not making sure she was dressed right and he just shrugged his shoulders and said, "Your Mummy can dress herself." She could dress herself, but she couldn't make good choices for the conditions or the occasion. More and more I was coming to the realization that Dad was not looking after Mom. He didn't want to. He didn't think to.

Going back to a few years earlier, I had accompanied my father on a three-week trip to India and Bangladesh because Mom didn't want to go. We were barely into the trip the first day, even at the airport, when Dad turned to me and patting his coat breast pocket and his pant pockets said, "Do you have the passports?" I panicked for a second, thinking he had forgotten or lost his. He found it and immediately passed it to me to keep. It was then I remembered all the trips we took with them and Mom kept everything until Dad needed it or asked for it. I felt like he was still a little boy needing his mother, but I also remembered that in India it was common for a man of some estate to have others to keep guard of their stuff. This was when I began to take over in ways I had seen my mother do for Dad and he immediately relaxed. Each time I saw him patting his coat or pants pocket I would say, "Dad. It's okay. I've got them."

He really depended on Mom all those years as a friend, companion, and personal secretary.

Good Gossip

People would tell me things about them when they saw me waiting for them in the entrance, or spending time with them in the common room having a snack and coffee. One lady told me that each evening after supper you could see them going for a walk on the grounds hand in hand and they all thought that was so lovely.

But another woman told me how Dad would go out through the doors first without paying attention to Mom following him and she was almost knocked over by the closing door several times. This I knew because I had chided him a few times in other places for not watching out for Mom right behind him. It was the rural Indian way for a woman to walk a few steps behind the man and I think Dad just got used to that when they were following the customs of the country they lived in for over twenty-five years.

I would try to visit them and check in at least twice a week. We had arranged for the phone number they had for years to be kept and installed in the Lodge. This meant that when people from out of town would come to visit Dad would call me to come over to the Lodge and entertain their guests. He obviously didn't know or understand the ways in which they could entertain guests using the facilities and services available.

They could register their guests to stay for the next meal and a special table would be provided. They could go down to the community kitchen and make coffee, tea, or hot chocolate with real creamers in the fridge. They could ask the main kitchen for cookies or treats baked that day and take them to where the guests were. These were designed and offered to help residents entertain visitors like they might in their own homes.

The one thing missing from their accommodations was a guest suite for staying overnight. Some of the facilities we had explored had a guest room like a hotel room you could book for your guests for a reasonable fee per night. The cleaning and bedding change would be done by the staff assigned to it.

We had a guest room I was ready to offer, but most of their out-of-town friends saw their situation and made other arrangements for their overnight stay. Many of them had stayed in Mom and Dad's home over the years. We were just happy they could at least have a short visit with friends who could see where they were living.

There were strict rules regarding the lockdown of the facility at night. All guests had to be out of the building by the time the front doors were locked. This was stressful for Dad whenever he wanted to take the car somewhere for a visit and had to worry about being back on time. If they missed supper they were chided by the management because if a resident wasn't present at the evening meal it was always investigated.

Mom didn't settle in at all and couldn't be out of sight of Dad without having a crying fit. Dad would point her to the elevator when he wanted to go out or visit and she wanted to go home. She would get to the elevator and then not know where to go or what to do. I think he was also a little embarrassed because all the other female residents knew where their rooms were, so why couldn't Mom figure it out too.

Dad soon realized he would have to escort her back to the room each time, pointing out the landmarks along the way to help her remember. Outside the doorway of each room was a little shelf. On that shelf were items each resident was encouraged to display to help them identify their rooms and guide visitors. Since they had two doors, we designated the door to the room they used as their living room as the main door. Each of them had a key on a lanyard to wear around their neck when they were out of their rooms. Mom had the key to the bedroom side, and Dad had the key to the living room side. This only made it more confusing for Mom and since she always needed help to find the room, having the familiar things on the outside didn't really help her know which floor they were on or what door to go into.

This situation progressed to the point where several times I went by and Mom was in the beauty salon having her hair done. Having it washed and set was something she did regularly because of her inability to lift her arms over her head to style her own hair. However, Dad began paying to have her hair permed within a couple of weeks of each other so he could have at least two hours on his own. When I realized what was happening, I just said, "Dad call me when you need to go out and I'll come over and stay with Mom but please don't give her any more perms for a couple of months at least!"

My brother Gary and his wife, Janice, recall visiting at the Lodge and suddenly seeing Mom come up to a window on the outside and wave at them. Dad didn't know where she was, didn't seem concerned, and Mom was just tickled to see them and came in for the visit. This seemed really strange to Gary and Janice. What was she doing outside?

One of the reasons Dad had chosen the Aspen Lodge as a place to live was because it was so close to his home church and he was often called on to lead chapel services there. They also had a couple of senior women who lived there and constantly remarked about how much they liked it. We thought that Dad would want to lead some of the chapels or make friends with the people they knew already in there and have them in to visit or play games with them and have coffee. None of that happened. Dad was so used to just leaving and going when and where he wanted to. He didn't mind leaving Mom home alone; because he thought she wouldn't go anywhere after that one incident when she got lost coming home. But as she began to wander in the Lodge, looking for him and asking after him, people began to take notice and mention these things to me. They weren't fitting in with the "swing" of the typical, normal, and daily lifestyle at the Lodge. And we didn't know the half of it, as it turned out.

Part of me wondered what they asked them in the interview, or what answers Mom and Dad had given them to make them believe they could be that independent and function with the level of "assistance" that was provided. With Christmas coming up, and seeing all the events and programs that were being planned, I ventured that it might help them feel more at home and figure out some of these things with a little help from others eager to have them as neighbors.

The Final Straw

As the Christmas season approached along with it came the flu. Mom got really sick and as was the facility's policy to avoid the spread of the virus, they would quarantine people in their rooms and bring their meals up on trays by staff.

So many residents were sick that they cancelled all the events, too much disappointment. But for Mom and Dad it was even worse than that. I visited Mom to see how she was doing, and she was dizzy, sick to her stomach, and not eating any of the delivered food. I made her a nice cup of tea in the community kitchen and sat with her. Dad in the meantime was staying as far away from her as possible and even spending the night in his recliner so he wouldn't get it.

I could see that she wasn't getting any care so I went down to the desk to talk to the manager on duty. I said, "Can I stay overnight to look after her?" And they said, "No. That is not allowed." I then asked, "What happens if she gets worse?" And they said, "We just call the ambulance." Visions of what happened to her when she had her surgery flashed through my mind. I said, "I can sleep in the recliner." But they said, "No. And you have to be out of here by the lockdown time." I went back to their suite with huge pain in my heart.

Part of me was angry at Dad for not being willing to care for her and for staying as far away from her as possible. Part of me was angry at our decision to think this would work for them. Most of me was angry because I wasn't allowed to stay and care for them and taking her home with me didn't seem like a good idea.

Dad promised me he would keep an eye on Mom and see that she got her medication for the night before he went to sleep. I felt he was a little mad about her condition and jealous for all the attention she was getting. He didn't mind the food being delivered to the room because then he didn't have to eat with their tablemate who sat bent over and never said anything. He was also looking forward to the Christmas choirs coming to entertain them and was blaming Mom for it being cancelled due to all the flu going around.

I prayed with them. Knelt by Mom's bed, smoothed her face, kissed her, and told her I would be back first thing in the morning. We prayed for God to take care of her and that she would not have to go to the hospital. I actually wondered how the staff would know if she was that much worse. If Dad was avoiding her and if she didn't have the presence of mind to pull one of the emergency cords, who would know? And that, strangely enough, gave me some comfort that she would still be there in the morning.

I got out of the building just as the doors were being locked and walked to my car. I got into the car and began to drive, but could hardly see the road. Tears spilled out of my eyes. My heart was breaking. I told God, "I don't know what to do. I just know they can't stay there any longer." I picked up my cell phone and called my sister. I burst out crying to the point that she thought one of them had died. When I finally was able to talk, I told her what was happening and that I couldn't take it anymore. We had to do something. Susie was all over it. "Do whatever you have to do. You have my support." I said, "Should we ask the boys?" And she said, "No, let's just make the best plan and let them know what and why." I didn't sleep all night for sitting up and listing all the pros and cons and what they really needed the most and what I would have to do to make it happen. I felt better and was at the door of the Lodge the minute they unlocked it for the day.

Thankfully Mom was better, and Dad ended up in bed having a better sleep than in the recliner. I stayed to make sure they had their breakfast, helped dress Mom and told them I was making plans to take them out of there. My search for a suitable place to rent began that very day. I put the word out and determined to find something as close to my own home as possible.

Linda McKendry

In spite of doing everything I could think of to make the transition to the Lodge easier and set up their space to accommodate what was most important to them, it wasn't the answer. I knew it was just a matter of time before another crisis. My plans to move them again didn't register with Mom. Dad had a look of bewilderment on his face as if it was both good news and bad news all at the same time. I was trying so hard to be respectful of him and honor him as my father, the "head"of our family, and Mom's ever-loving husband, but I realized I had to "take the bull by the horns" and at least explore some options. God answered our prayers, as you will see in the next chapters.

They had a holiday planned for a couple of weeks away to stay with friends they had known from one of their churches. The timing was such that after giving notice in writing they would be gone when we had to move them out. It didn't seem like the best idea for transition of people with dementia, but I had no choice and was not going to leave them there for another month.

When I went in to the Lodge's office to officially give the notice of vacating, they wanted to know why. Most residents only moved out because they died, or had to be transferred to a facility for round-the-clock care requiring nursing or special equipment. For every objection I had regarding things like the laundry, non-compliance on medication, etc. they would say, "Well, we can hire someone to do that. We can hire someone to do that." And I said, "Who are you going to hire to stay by my Mom's bedside all night when she needs it?" I told them we appreciated all they wanted to do and the wonderful staff they had there, but in order to keep them together and care for them in the way we had promised them we needed to take them out.

I distinctly remember carrying the big brown envelope with all the contracts and details of their rental along with a copy of the letter of notice and thinking, "I'm taking them out of boarding school!" It made me feel good that what I had wanted for years at boarding school in Northern India, I was able to make happen for them.

Finding More Evidence

My niece and I went to clean out their room after the movers had packed up their furniture. The floors and window ledges looked like they had not been vacuumed or dusted in all the time they had been there. I don't blame the staff because the residents were supposed to put items up if they wanted surfaces cleaned.

The one time I tried to be there on the room cleaning day, I found that Mom had lined the waste basket in their bathroom with one of her pull-ups and not the used plastic grocery bags I had collected for that purpose.

We found pills everywhere. I already knew that Dad's medication was out of compliance by three months and Mom's was non-compliant for two. I felt a huge wave of guilt come over me for not monitoring it other than wondering why they had so many stacks of medication packs. I just assumed the pharmacist had sent over what they needed ahead of time.

We also found a lot of cookies wrapped in paper napkins tucked in here and there that Mom had obviously brought up from the 8:00 pm snack times. She didn't want to eat them but didn't know what to do with them. I could imagine her saying "No thank you!" and Dad urging, "Come on Lydia, you need the energy." Dad never turned down free food!

Linda McKendry

Because of a single hole in the wall behind Dad's chair where we had hung a picture as we were told we could, we were not refunded the full damage deposit and it felt just like one more reason I didn't want to be there anymore.

I must say that the last thing I did was to stand in the full sunlight and look out the window of their little living room. They faced south and got nice light and sun all day facing the north side of the Calgary Zoo on St. George's Island. There was a beautiful view of green lawn breaking up the parking lot and the tall mature trees across one of the main roads into the downtown core of Calgary that was always quiet after rush hour.

It just went to show that no matter how beautiful the view, the accommodations, the finishes on the floors, walls, and lighting or the high-quality furnishings and accessories, if you aren't well in your body, soul or your spirit, you can't enjoy it at all. All that remained was to see how they would adjust to the new home we had prepared for them and how we could take care of them.

LIFE AFTER THE LODGE

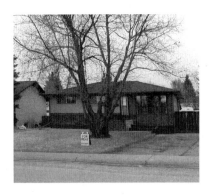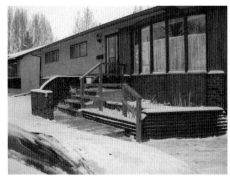

The House and A Half

<u>The House:</u> We kept our promise to Mom and Dad that if it wasn't working at the Aspen Lodge Assisted Living facility, we would take them out. Of course the house they had lived in for many years had been sold. The cash equity topped up their nest egg so we had options for their care. Bringing them home meant finding a new suitable house for them to live in. This was the closest we could come to our original promise.

The wonderful market in which we had sold their home, however, now had a downside for finding a home to rent. Choices were extremely limited and rents really high. My prime need was for a house closer to me and one that was a bungalow with only a few stairs, if any. I was also on the lookout for a house that might work for me to move them and my consulting business into. The search was on, with much prayer.

My daughter called to say that there was a little bungalow for rent across the road from where she was taking her children to school. She lived just a few blocks away. She said it had recently been the headquarters for one of the parties during a civic election and had been vacant for a while. I called and found out what the rent was. It was in the budget if we combined what Mom and Dad were paying per month at the Lodge and what I was paying in the commercial space I rented. The only catch was the amount of cash needed for the first and last rent, as the damage deposit.

I didn't have that amount of cash handy, so I looked around at what I could liquidate and my eyes fell on my baby grand piano. I checked into prices for used grands online and put it on Kijiji for sale at the amount of cash I needed. Before I could even get any responses, I told my sister what I was doing and why. She offered to purchase the piano, have it shipped to their home in BC because she loves to play and always imagined having a beautiful grand piano. That was a win-win and soon I was looking in the vacant house near Kim to determine where everything could fit in. The extra benefit was that before being used as the campaign headquarters the landlord had his mortgage brokerage business there, so ample lines were already installed for phones, faxes, and modems.

Since Mom and Dad had just spent several months living in two adjoining rooms at the lodge with trips to the dining room and common activity room, I decided we could set them up in the three bedrooms on one side of the house. I chose the largest bedroom, with the double closet to become the master bedroom. It was right across the hall from the bathroom past a built-in linen closet. In the next room, adjacent to the bathroom, I set up a little den. It was right around the corner from the washroom so Mom would easily find it when she stepped out of the den.

Susie came and helped me make choices for better sized furnishings because what we had taken from their home to the

Lodge were on a larger scale and too big to fit into the space properly. In some ways it was another downsizing, but this time we invested in pieces more suitable. We furnished this room with a wall mounted TV shelf, their recliner chairs, table, lamp, coordinating area rug, and a fold out couch that made into a bed. This meant that friends and family could stop by and have a nice little visit with them in this space. It was also a place for me to sleep overnight if needed, and it was close to them and the washroom. We believed they would like our choices since they were more to their taste than ours.

The third bedroom was where we set up Dad's clock repair shop. It increased his workshop and wall display space by four times what they had in the Lodge. This room was right around the corner from the front entrance, so customers wouldn't have to go through the entire house. Mom could hang out in the den within ear shot of Dad doing business, which she was used to for years.

Across from this room was the kitchen and since Dad always liked to offer coffee and cookies to his guests or customers, I felt this would work for him too.

This house had a sun porch off of a cement patio so there was a place for all of us to enjoy sitting in the sun all year round. The basement had a two-bedroom suite and a full bathroom so I felt that was either a good place for visiting family and friends to stay or I could rent it out for extra income. I also knew that if we had a live-in nurse that would be her living quarters. This all felt like it was a good solution to all the things we wanted and needed at that time.

Also, I had decided that the back door would be ideal for them to use for their entrance because it had a more spacious entrance before going up a couple of steps into the kitchen. It had a much larger closet for coats, boots, canes, umbrellas and other things. I knew there was power in precedent and had intended to take them into that entrance the first time we brought them there. However, that isn't what happened. The day they moved in Dad was already making his way up the front steps with Mom in tow and it didn't feel right to turn them around and make them go into the back. They never did use the back entrance. This was their home, was the reminder.

The Half: The living-dining room would be my office, consultation room, and space for filing cabinets and storage units. The kitchen then became the common eating space as the place for their main meals. It also served as a "staff room" for me for coffee and entertaining clients who occasionally came to my office. I had an assistant who was part time and did mostly data entry and filing. My business also rented the garage, and I put down a false floor to cover all the car oil stains to use it for my studio. This all happened in the spring so even though the garage wasn't heated, I decided not to worry about that until winter set in. This was my business.

This meant that going to my office each day also allowed me to step into their world and keep an eye on them. I felt like the killing of the two proverbial birds each day was going to work. It also meant that I could plan, prepare, and make sure they were eating well and on time with dinner on the table for them before I went home to my husband each evening.

I reasoned that since no one had put them to bed each night at the Lodge they would be capable of getting themselves ready for bed, having their evening prayers which was their habit, and being a phone call away if they had an emergency. With Kim just around the block, I knew I could call on her to run over and be there quickly while I was on my way. We believed we had everything covered, and most importantly, they were together.

Confusion Reigns

I felt that my job was to figure out how to make things work for them, but it didn't take long to find out what worked and what didn't. I have a saying, "I'm not a slave to my house or my possessions. They are slaves to me." And while it was a house and a half depending on who needed the most space, it was always a whole house in our hearts for what we were doing.

We don't know to this day if it was a mistake to move their stuff and change up their familiar furnishings while they were on an extended road trip to visit friends. But that's the way it worked out. It kept them together. Safe. Sound. And Sane! Or so I thought.

The first incident was a sewer backup in the basement the day after we moved them in. The foul odor was the first clue. I checked it out and called the landlord who came over immediately. The city came to scope the sewer lines and found two things had caused the problem. First, because the house has been vacant for so many months there hadn't been any water to flush the drains and keep them clean. Raw sewage, toilet paper, and what appeared to be Kleenex had plugged the drain and hardened. Secondly, the city found some of the clay sewer pipe had been broken by the roots of the mature trees in the yard. An auger was used to clear everything out of the way to get it all flowing again. Fortunately, the yard didn't have to be dug up and all the sewer drainage pipes replaced.

The landlord had to remove the entire floor covering in the basement and have a crew come in and sanitize the areas where any backup touched walls or doors. In the meantime Mom and

Linda McKendry

Dad came to stay in my home until the house was a safe and functional environment for them.

Even though they had visited our home a few times in Toronto, they had never had any cause to stay overnight with us in Calgary. My stepson had stopped in overnight and was sleeping soundly on a couch just outside their room. In the morning when I came down to check on them, I found them, fully dressed, laying on the bed, terrified! They were so glad to see me.

Dad said, "We didn't know where we were." Mom said, "I looked outside and there's a guard sleeping on the couch so we were too afraid to leave the room and look for you." I felt terrible but immediately invited them upstairs and made their favorite breakfast which relaxed everyone. They were understandably confused about everything and I couldn't wait to take them to the house, especially since that was now also my office and I had projects to look after.

In a few days we were back in their home and the suite in the basement had all new floor coverings and felt fresh and clean. We had confidence too that the sewage system was working even though we were warned not to flush wipes or facial tissue down the toilet. Life, I felt, would settle into a routine and things would become familiar.

They were confused at first when they stepped into my office in the living-dining room. It was a constant reminder to them of what we had done and why we had moved again. Several times Dad talked as if he was back in their old house, asking me to go downstairs and bring up something for him from under the stairs. He also expressed suspicions about missing tools and equipment from his clock shop and I had to remind him that he had sold or donated them to his clock club buddies. I just kept praying for them to feel safe and at home. Each time I saw Mom reach over to touch Dad's arm and smile at him or pass their bedroom where they slept together surrounded by the furniture they had used for years, I felt good.

The Wake-Up Calls

I had to accept the fact that Dad was not looking after Mom at the Lodge and the results were that they were both feeling lost. I didn't know if what we had arranged was going to work and I too felt lost for a moment. I took them on a little tour and they began to see all their familiar personal things in the bathroom and bedroom. The little den we had arranged for them they saw was comfortable, but not familiar at all. The kitchen was stocked with pots and pans, dishes, and baking equipment my daughter got from her friend whose grandma had lived with them and recently passed away.

After getting rid of all these things when we downsized, we joked about having to go to the Good Will stores and buy them back. We felt like the gift from Kim's friend was a windfall and she was happy that her grandma's things were going to make the lives of Kim's grandparents better. Dad even thought that the pattern name on the bottom of the dishes which was "Vibe" was a sign because at that time he was still driving his Pontiac Vibe! Little things like that popped up to make us feel more at home and help us all move forward.

Because we had downsized Dad's shop to fit into a little corner in their bedroom at the Lodge, he really felt like a lot of stuff was missing now that the room was so much larger and very vacant looking. He was fixated on a lathe that he said he needed, and we knew it had gone to one of the clock club members. Even though he would nod in agreement each time we reminded him, he was still on the lookout for it. Often, he would go down to the basement or send Mom to look "under the stairs" for things that had been stored there in their original home. These were the signs to me that they didn't know where things had gone.

I resorted to what they had gotten used to by combining what they were doing in their original home and at the Lodge. At the lodge they were eating three meals a day and three snacks in between at specific times and that seemed to be what they had gotten used to. In their original home they had also survived for a time on the Meals on Wheels program. So, I scoured the supermarket for nourishing frozen dinners that they could share, making sure desserts of biscuits and fruit cups were included. I felt this would be a timesaving way of preparing meals for them with my busy work schedule.

I would get Mom to help me set the table so she could feel useful, keep moving, and become familiar with things in the kitchen. Like directing a child, as long as I pointed out each step, she was okay to do it. I had to say, "The plates are right over there, Mom, on that shelf. We just need the middle size ones." She didn't move to put them out on her own. I would heat up the meals, call them to the table, and serve them, put out the desserts and often have to leave with instructions for their snacks at 8 pm and their bedtime reminder. Medications were given at this mealtime too.

Dad always knew what time it was and had the schedule firmly fixed in his mind. He would remind us if it was five and he hadn't been called to the table. We never chided him and just calmed him down by saying it was almost ready... or he could come to the table and wait if he wanted to.

Done With Dementia

Two incidents happened soon after that that made me realize they were not safe to be left alone and we had to increase the level of care to around the clock. The first was when I decided to go into my office one evening. It was around nine. I knew that if they were in bed, they would have just gone there. I was surprised to see the light on in the kitchen and walked in on them having "breakfast." I said, "What are you guys doing?" Dad said, "We must have slept in. We woke up and realized it was after eight so we got up to make breakfast." I asked, "When did you go to bed?" He said, "Last night." I said, "Dad, this is last night and it's 9 o'clock in the evening not tomorrow morning." He looked a little sheepish and I could clearly see he didn't know what to do or say. Since our Canadian winters are dark very early in the evening and still dark later in the morning, he had become confused. I decided that either stopping by or calling in more often was what I needed to do.

The next incident is very difficult for me to share. I feel I need to because that is what our story is all about. I once again stopped in to check on them and heard the shower on in the bathroom and Mom crying out, "Johnny, it's cold!" I walked in to find Mom standing naked in the tub supporting herself with her hands against the wall. Dad was standing on the outside of the tub hosing her down with the hand-held shower. I said, "What's going on? What are you doing, Dad?" He replied without even stopping, "Lydia has dung all over her rear and I'm washing her off."

I immediately took over by turning the water off, throwing a towel over Mom and letting Dad dry his hands so he could leave the bathroom. She looked so helpless and confused. She was shivering, she was still soiled, and the tub needed to be rinsed as well. I threw a towel on the floor and helped her step out onto it. She was worried about soiling it. "Mom, it can be washed. It's no big deal."

I ran some warm water and used a washcloth to gently clean her off, dry her, and find her night clothes.

When everything was settled, she would so often say, "Thank you, darling." Dad was usually just quiet, working on one of his word search puzzles. I said, "Dad, from now on please just ask me to help her. I don't mind, really!" The way he was treating her in the tub made me think of him as a boy, back on the farm, hosing down a cow or a horse. He refused to use the word, "shit" and we were greatly reprimanded for using it, so I guess the word "dung" was acceptable. We began to use the words "pee", "poop" and "potty" many times a day to deal with the incontinence issues. This was also when I decided that having nice fitting under garments for Mom to wear that didn't leak or have an odor would be at the top of my list of well stocked supplies. I knew I wanted to make this house into a "happy home" and work out all the details of what they needed. Each time a little crisis surfaced I took it in stride and made necessary adjustments, and each change put us in a better place to keep things calm and comfortable.

Expanding Their Space

So, while the house was set up and functional in every way, we faced two problems. I knew that they wouldn't really feel at home until they had the living room back and could sit and look out the front bay window (the bedroom windows were halfway up the wall in their den.) It was in the fall of 2008 that the bottom fell out of the economy and it affected my business. I regrouped and solicited some other business to fill the gap, including giving seminars and workshops in the community center next to the school across the road. The potential was huge, and the prospects were great, but it put more stress on my time too.

Done With Dementia

It was around this time that Dad was hospitalized. Our funds hadn't come in yet from the Self Managed Funding, and I missed a deadline for writing an article for the first time in my life. I didn't have a cushion of time or money and didn't have the support in place either. We had just secured the services of a foreign worker nurse, Sol, from the Philippines who was living downstairs.

I decided that taking care of Mom and Dad was my main mandate. I closed my consulting business of eighteen years. This meant that I no longer needed all the office space or conference tables. I reduced my workspace into the dining area and moved what was in the den into the living room. The den was turned into the caregiver's bedroom.

I also cleaned out the garage and took my studio supplies back to my house and rearranged my own basement storage room to organize it for that purpose. This also saved us some money since I had been renting the garage separately. Dad often complained that his car was parked in the front driveway when he looked out and saw the garage in the back. At one time the landlord also had a couple of vacation trailers parked in the back yard until I asked him to move them so we could mow the lawn properly. That also caused less confusion for Dad when he looked out into the back yard.

In the living room I arranged their chairs, so they were facing the window. Mom and Dad immediately perked up. They loved watching the babies and toddlers on the swings waiting for preschoolers to get out of school at the community center. In the winter they watched the skaters on the outdoor rink and the school kids making snow huts and snowmen during recess. The davenport that made into a bed was moved into the living room as a couch and extra bed when needed. When friends and family came to visit it was much more like home, and Dad was quick to place his order to whoever was in the kitchen for coffee or snacks.

I looked at the house as just space available for whatever we needed at the time. Each room morphed in those first few months until we settled into the layout that worked best for everyone. Routine was established and every detail was organized so each caregiver knew what to do and where to find what was needed.

It boiled down to just making sure we had the right people in place at the right time so no one, including me, would suffer burnout. I was always on the lookout for responsible people, friends or acquaintances of Mom and Dad's, who I felt comfortable asking for some help in ways that would be easy and comfortable for them. When extra funds were available, I could offer to pay for a nice lunch or dinner out with Mom and Dad as an outing for them and some respite for us.

The Leaky Bucket
That Almost Got Kicked

<u>Dad's Crisis:</u> Taking Mom and Dad to their regular checkups and medical appointments helped me to know their medical conditions and explain symptoms to the doctor. Their family GP was Dr. Yee. Both Mom and Dad had seen him for years and it helped that his office was in a professional space on the second floor of a big indoor shopping center. This meant that parking was always free and ample and we could plan coffee times and lunch around the food court as part of a nice outing.

Before they went into the Aspen Lodge, they joked that they weren't going to go for annual checkups anymore because they could always find something wrong at their age. They explained that by the time they went for all the tests, diagnostics, and referrals to specialists, and got the prescribed medication or therapy, it was time for their next checkup! They decided that they would only call a doctor if they had some chronic symptoms or an emergency, like a fall or cut.

Dad's blood tests, over several checkups, continued to reveal that he had really low iron. I asked the doctor if an iron supplement would solve the problem. Dr. Yee thought doing that would be like filling a bucket that had a leak in it and he wanted to get to the real problem: where the blood loss was. He suggested that we get an MRI. At that time the wait times for this new technology was very long and Dad's condition wasn't considered life threatening. However, my doctor brother-in-law decided to pay for Dad to have an MRI in a private clinic, which we did ASAP. We were somewhat relieved that nothing showed up on that test. However,

Linda McKendry

as the low iron in blood tests continued to show a "leak" as Dr. Yee called it, we needed to step up the diagnostics. Dr. Adrianna Cohen, a gerontologist on the faculty at the University Hospital looked over the reports from Dr. Yee and ordered a CT scan. If we were willing to drive to a nearby town we could get the tests done more quickly.

I still remember the day I drove Dad down. Mom was content to stay home with Sol, our nurse. As we sat in the waiting area filling out the form, I had to ask Dad for answers to the questions like, "What did your mother die from?" Dad answered, "Old age." "What did your father die from?" Same answer, "Old age." I just laughed as I kept filling in this answer. I knew that his mother, my grandma Gamble, suffered severe symptoms of abdominal pain, because the last time I had visited her in the nursing home, I left her room in tears. I couldn't handle the pain she was in. Dad didn't remember any of that. I also thought of how there was a day when people just died of "Old Age" because we didn't have so many specific conditions or diseases labelled.

This CT scan revealed that there was a tumor, a mass in Dad's large intestine. The good news was that it appeared to be self-contained and had not spread into surrounding organs, like the liver. We were referred to Dr. Buie, the surgeon who had supervised Mom's surgery on her bowel prolapse repair. After examining Dad and looking at the diagnostics he ordered a colonoscopy. He said that was necessary to actually take a look at the tumor to plan the surgery. He also said that not having the surgery risked the tumor growing and blocking the intestine which would be extremely painful and require emergency surgery. At that point it might also spread to other organs and become a full-blown fatal cancer case.

I remember taking Dad into the hospital for this test. Dad was in a gown and on a gurney ready to be wheeled into the diagnostics room. We had followed the protocol to clean out the bowel and other than his morning medication with a little water, he wasn't allowed to eat or drink. Since he was looking forward to his first cup of coffee of the day, I decided to store his clothes and shoes in a locker, take his wallet with me and head down to the hospital cafeteria and bring back a take-out coffee.

I barely got out of the room when I saw the orderly wheeling him back. I quickly returned to get his clothes out of the locker and help him dress. I was stopped by a doctor holding a file which he opened up to show me a beautiful full color image of a large marble size black tumor on the side of a very healthy-looking wall of Dad's colon. As it turned out, the minute they sent the scope into the colon, it showed up, so they took the picture and Dad was done!

The doctor said it appeared to be totally contained and would be quick and easy for Dr. Buie to remove. I shared this information with Dad and the family. Dad seemed reluctant to go ahead, because he didn't feel any discomfort at the time. We kept remembering that Dr. Buie told us what the risks would be if we didn't do anything and it grew. We explained this to Dad while he nodded as if he heard and understood. Being his enduring power of attorney, I knew I had the legal right and authority to make this decision. I chose to go ahead. Dr. Buie's office called to give us pre-surgical instructions and scheduled the day.

On the way to the hospital the day of surgery we were caught in traffic because of an accident. It was winter and the roads were icy. I called the hospital to let them know we were on our way but might be late. They said we had lots of time. I asked Dad how he was feeling about it all. He immediately said, "I'm not worried. I've lived a good life and I'm ready to go if I don't make it." I signed off the DNR order, which is "Do Not Resuscitate." We had discussed this with Dr. Yee for their Life Capsule in the fridge if EMS had to come into their home. I just followed that directive.

Dr. Buie said it would be a "classic" short procedure. He gave me his direct line to call when the patient tracking monitor in the visitor's lounge showed Dad in the recovery room. We watched as each patient scheduled that day went through all the stages of their surgical procedures. When the time came, Dr. Buie was happy to tell me that everything went just as planned. He also said, "We got it all and took 15 cm of the bowel, which was the blood system for it. He won't need any radiation or chemotherapy." That was such a relief and I praised God for this good news.

After experiencing Mom's melt down due to her dementia after her bowel surgery, we planned to schedule a family "vigil" to help Dad in his recovery in the hospital. Dr. Cohen had authorized us to be there 24/7 due to his dementia, so the medical team accepted this. The first challenge with Dad after surgery was his reluctance to move as much as they wanted him to. Helping him into the washroom was the most frequent task, and he seemed to be progressing as expected. On the fourth day, one of the staff was particularly assertive with him. My sister was on duty with him at the time and she was very concerned at the level of pressure being used on Dad. He collapsed. His heart had stopped, and he wasn't breathing. The calls went out on the PA and the blue cart was ordered. Suddenly someone got Susie's attention to ask if they could resuscitate him, and she said "Yes!" She either didn't know or remember that we had signed off on a DNR. God took over that decision anyways as his heart began to beat on its own before the cart even got there. It was a good sign. So they gave him oxygen and moved him down to ICU.

Dr. Buie had said that Dad needed to take it easy while the incision on the bowel healed and that if it did "tear" emergency surgery would be necessary and it could mean an ileostomy bag to empty. In terms of caregiving we didn't want this. Now there was no choice. The worst had to be faced. Imagine my surprise when I came to the hospital to take my turn with him and walked into a hospital room that was empty, including the unmade bed! I was quickly sent down to ICU where Susie was next to a wheelchair piled with all Dad's personal clothes, his favorite pillow, and his slippers.

The shock was seeing him listless and hooked up to so many tubes. He was also on a breathing machine and it didn't look good. He was scheduled for the emergency surgery.

He had suffered from septic shock, which meant that his body was full of the toxins and "waste" designed to be eliminated through the intestines and colon. Susie was feeling a little bad that she had made the call to resuscitate Dad, but also as grateful as I was, that God had stepped in to cause Dad's heart to start on its own. This alone gave us a lot of hope for a good outcome.

We spoke with Dr. Buie and he said there was a treatment available for someone his age in this serious a condition. It could only be given for 48 hours and it was known to be effective and the side effects were "rare but fatal." He needed to know in about twenty minutes whether to go ahead or not. Dr. Buie had come in to the visitor's lounge to explain this option. We immediately had a family meeting. My daughter, Kim, leaned over to him before he left and asked, "If that was your grandpa out there suffering from this, would you give him the treatment?" To which he replied, "Yes." I think we wanted the guarantee of at least another 48 hours. Susie went around the room, like a contestant judge, "Linda? Yes or no?" "Eldon, yes or no?" "Gary, yes or no?" It was a unanimous "yes," and I assumed she agreed with the popular vote, even though she never expressed her opinion. I was sent to find Dr. Buie and tell him we had agreed to the treatment. He also went ahead to do the necessary repair surgery and install a stoma for attaching to an external ileostomy bag.

We had told the medical team we were a family of faith. We were prepared for the worst, but expected the best. We did everything to be respectful and cooperative with the medical team.

I stood on one side of Dad's bed and my brothers were on the other. I said, "I'm going to pray a prayer, make declarations and all you have to do is agree with me." I listed the four things they had said were wrong with Dad. I declared his heart stable, his lungs clear, his body free from infection, and his kidneys functioning, and added, "In the name of Jesus!" That was it.

The next morning, we were surprised to find that Dad had been taken off the oxygen because he began to breathe on his own during the night. His heart was strong and regular. By the following day we came in to find him sitting up with a suction wand he was told to spit into whenever he coughed. He had been taken off the treatment because his condition wasn't deemed severe enough.

He had been on some strong opioids and was hallucinating. He saw his grey slippers as two big rats under the bed and the light on the wall as the moon coming up. But he was such a joker all the time that we didn't really know if he was seeing things or just being funny. Our prayers and anointing with oil were witnessed by others in emergency and they began to come over and ask us to come and pray for their loved ones. My sister is a certified Chaplain so we knew she could operate in that capacity without any offense.

Dad was in ICU for ten days and then stable enough to move up to a recovery ward. We were given a lounge chair that made into a flat bed so we could take turns staying with Dad and helping him 24/7. There were times when he needed help to use the urinal and because of the ileostomy bag, which the nurses or orderly changed; he would never need the toilet again for his bowel. As each of us watched the procedure and asked questions we were getting trained to help Dad when he was released.

That was thirty-seven days later and he had lost so much weight that we had to bring in clothes that fit his new frame. He wasn't eating, so Dr. Buie told us he was going to take him off the hospital food and we could bring in anything he would eat. It took a good feed of East Indian takeout food to kick start his appetite as we met in the cafeteria the first time he was out of his room. We also made toast with butter, peanut butter and honey in the ward kitchen for frequent snacks along with coffee.

I was there the day they brought in a therapist to test him for standing and walking. He almost collapsed in the arms of the therapist! He had been bedridden too long and was very weak. They recommended a ten-day stay at the Geriatric Recovery Department in a hospital really close to their home. After his first week there we could bring him home for a visit, and if I made the decision he could stay home and not return.

Linda McKendry

The therapists there pleaded with me to make him come back for one more week. He had to be able to walk fifteen steps with a cane or walker and do five stairs before they considered him strong enough to go home. He was so delighted with all the attention of these two wonderful ladies that his progress was amazing for the first week. They felt that if he progressed as far in the second week as in the first, he would really be on the way to full recovery. It was hard to make the decision because he wanted to stay home after that first visit. But I talked him into going back for one more week. Then we were given exercises to do that would keep him getting stronger by the day.

We had a raised bungalow so there were the five stairs to the front outside from the sidewalk, and on bad days, we had the five stairs down to the back-entrance landing. While he grumbled and complained, he still cooperated and even got on his stationary bike as long as he could. All we had to do was to feed him, increase milk to cream for cereal and coffee, and two pieces of toast instead of one at breakfast. It wasn't long before we had to cut back and slow the weight gain! One of the hospital staff happened to see my Dad's name come across her screen, so she checked to see what he was in for. She told me later that it was his weight that saved his life as reserve energy he needed for a crisis like that. Who knew?

Mom's Reaction to Dad's Crisis

We had been bringing Mom in every day to visit Dad. When I came on duty, I would take Sol, our nurse, to be with Dad during the day so the staff could see that we had a full-time nurse and be more confident to let him come home sooner. Mom was then seeing Dad each morning and each afternoon when I did this shift change. Mom got along with Sol and they would sit and laugh together a lot. Sol called her "Mom" and she responded, even with polite gratitude, but never any requests for help of any kind.

When Dad was still in ICU, Susie had taken Mom with the nurse to the Shopping Mall that was famous for a big carrousel. I had taken Mom there numerous times and she loved to ride the horses while Dad sat at a table nearby with a coffee and his puzzle book. She was like a little kid and the operator said she wasn't the only old lady who loved to ride the horses. Susie had called to see if she should bring Mom in to see Dad. We weren't sure because he was hooked up to so many tubes and wires.

There were ten beds in this acute emergency room and Dad was in the second one as you came in the door. But you had to pass the first one, which was partially glassed in, in which there was a man who was suffering third degree burns. He looked awful and I was worried that Mom would think that was Dad and react with shock. We decided as a family that Mom should come and see Dad, but I warned Susie about the condition of the man in the first bed. I suggested she distract Mom as they rounded the corner to Dad's bed or explain quickly that wasn't Dad. When Susie arrived at the ICU, I was watching out for her and anxious to see how she would react to Dad. We pulled up a chair for her next to Dad's bed. She looked him up and down, sat in the chair, patted him on the part of his arm sticking out from the gown that didn't have a needle or tape stuck to it and said, "Johnny. I was just riding a beautiful horse. It was white. And there was a brown one and a black one..." We stood there with big smiles on our faces because she sounded so sincere and looked so cute.

Since she had a family member around all the time, mostly my sister Susie, the only thing she needed to know was, "Where's my Johnny?" When we said, "He's in the hospital, Mom," she would say, "When's he coming home?" And if we told her what had happened to him, it was as if she was hearing it for the first time so we began to make light of it and focus on taking her for a visit, or tell her he'd be home "tomorrow" if it was evening. If we gave her an answer, she seemed all right for the moment until she thought to ask again in a few minutes. The usual distractions of turning on her favorite musical groups helped a bit, but each time she sat at the table and Dad wasn't there, she would have to ask again. It was hard.

Dad's first visit from the Geriatric Recovery Department was on her birthday, so we were happy that he could at least celebrate that with her, even though my brothers had to practically carry him up the front stairs due to his weakness. This was when I decided to make him go back to the recovery unit for another week. It was worth it in the long run. But she never commented on Dad's weight loss, or all the tubes he was attached to in the hospital. She would just hold his hand if he'd let her or pat his arm and you could see her contentment at just being next to him. Those were the times I was so happy to have them together with the freedom to take her back and forth as many times as we wanted to see Dad daily.

While he was in hospital and not walking yet, my sister-in-law, Ruth, who volunteered at the MCC Thrift Shop called to say they had a working hospital bed for $400. I asked her to put a hold on it and checked it out immediately. Jim had just purchased a larger truck and was able to transport it and get it into the house with the help of my brothers. It was very heavy and awkward. What a Godsend. Someone else had given us a hospital table and this was used to display all the supplies needed to change Dad's ileostomy bag once a week after his shower.

Done With Dementia

This extra care and attention Dad needed came from Sol, the nurse, when she was on duty and Mom was unable to understand what she was doing to Dad when he was naked to the groin or when they were in the bathroom together. When Mom stood in the doorway or approached Dad's bed when Sol was treating him, Dad would shoo her away. She began to hover just outside in the hallway. From that time on, she didn't like the nurse. She would call her names and tell her she was stupid and "naughty." We could understand why, but we couldn't make her understand and from then on Mom couldn't be left alone with Sol without Dad around to keep Mom calm.

Things regressed in the next few years even when we had a different nurse. We had some overnight issues with Mom, and I ended up having to spend each night in the caregiver's room. When the nurse was on duty overnight, she slept in the hospital bed, but after a while I just let her go home to the apartment she shared with others from her country. We had to put the hospital bed table across the hall so Mom wouldn't wander into the other parts of the house. The couple of times she had done this, she had gotten confused and in one case fell on the stairs in the sunroom and fractured some ribs. The nurse tried to coax her back, but she wouldn't cooperate. It was at that time we also put a latch high on the back door to the stairs.

I am sharing these things so that you, dear reader, can learn from some of the things we went through and some of the areas where we could have been more proactive. Because Mom was still getting up at night to use the washroom, we didn't want to give her too much sleeping aid. We felt that would contribute to a fall, so we didn't anticipate she would wander down into the back of the house in the dark. The following day I also had to clean the soiled floor in the sunroom, so it appeared she was trying to find the bathroom because her bowel was loose. That too had never happened before. She usually just peed in the middle of the night.

I felt so bad for her and could only imagine how shocked she must have been when she missed that one step into the sunporch. It's no different than having a child for whom you want to do everything and make sure they are always safe and sound. You feel terrible when something goes wrong that you know you could have possibly prevented. But this too is part of our story. Each time we encountered a crisis or something we hadn't anticipated; we quickly made the changes necessary to prevent it from happening again.

Dad's recovery and caregiving by the nurse triggered Mom to not like or want to cooperate with the nurses, which made it challenging for me personally as I was the one who picked up the slack. I began to spend every night at the house and sleep there, going home during the day when the nurse came on duty.

Topping Up the Piggy Bank

Win-Win Income

Not knowing how long they would live or how long we would need to care for them meant that I was being very budget conscious with all the available funds. Even at that I felt the pinch and decided to either rent out the second bedroom downstairs for someone to share that space with the nurse, or to take advantage of the school and offer afterschool care. The YMCA had closed down the afterschool care service and I knew several working parents were looking around for options in the neighborhood.

I created one of those tear off ads you see on public bulletin boards and took it over to the school office across the road where my grandchildren went to school. The staff were very positive especially when they could look across the playground to the house I pointed to when I explained our situation. I did some research and decided that our fee for afterschool care would be $400 a month, based on parents working nine to five, or ten to six in retail. The nurse would be on duty when the kids would be needing care. In addition to her parents, our foreign nurse was supporting a very young son, back home in the Philippines. We knew she really missed him, calling each day, and sending back packages like my Mom did for us when we were in boarding school in India. She seemed to enjoy the company of my grandchildren. She was quick to fix them snacks, offer them goodies, and play with them. They loved her too.

I then called the Home Care Coordinator and told her that if she knew of a senior who was mobile enough for the stairs and needed a place to live, we had an extra room in a nicely finished two-bedroom suite. I explained that because we had 24/7 care and were already making meals and doing housekeeping, we felt some senior could take advantage of our situation at a very reasonable cost, with very little extra work for us. I told her the room and board would be $500 a month. I knew some basement suites were renting for $750 a month, so this seemed reasonable for me since the space had to be shared.

On the very same day, I had the home care supervisor bring Joe, a senior, over to look at the accommodation in the basement and a couple came by with their child for afterschool care. While I had thought I could only do one or the other, it turned out, once again, that by arranging furniture and organizing the space we could do both.

Linda McKendry

Joe and Adan: Joe moved in right away. He was handsome, healthy, and had owned and operated a car repair garage for years. He had cared for his wife who passed away after several years of needing 24/7 care. He had a triple bypass and his family had believed he would die from it and sold his house and most of his possessions. In a miracle turn of events, he had survived and now because of his dementia, which was very mild, he had been unable to sign off to make anyone his enduring power of attorney. He had a daughter who visited and took him out from time to time and I made sure to keep her in the loop regarding any of his needs or his condition. He brought a few possessions like a favorite chair, side tables and TV. We supplied his bed, chest of drawers, and linens. He shared the washroom, kitchen, and table and chairs with the nurse.

Joe needed help remembering his medication, but he was very strong and sturdy with no issues for the stairs. He ate whatever we prepared for Mom and Dad and seemed genuinely happy to have our home as his home. He was willing to shovel snow in the winter and mow the lawn in the summer for which we were paid by Dad's Veterans Affairs allowance. I passed this on to Joe for a little extra pocket money. Each time we went out, we would invite Joe to come along and he sat in the back seat with Mom who doted on him and made him feel really special, while she kept an eye on Dad in the front seat. Joe was always there to help take Mom's arm and help her over a curb or hold the door open for Dad. The kids loved him too.

Joe was often on his own on weekends. He liked to walk to nearby eateries or take the bus to visit friends or family. While his daughter and I both worried a little that he might get lost one day due to dementia, he had his cell phone and used it. He didn't use the stove or do any cooking downstairs, like Sol did. But he had an electric kettle to make a quick tea, coffee or hot chocolate. The nurse was a little uncomfortable at first sharing the bathroom, but I organized the space so that their personal items were separate.

I also had a lock installed on her door and told her she could use Mom and Dad's bathroom if she wanted to. Joe turned out to be an angel in disguise and was always offering to help with all sorts of things. Joe referred to our parents as "Mom" and "Dad," never John and Lydia. I really appreciated having him and it was a "win-win" for all of us: a "Godsend."

Adan was in one of the lower grades. He was an only child. His dad was a tradesman in the construction industry and usually was at work really early so his mother, who worked regular hours at a print shop, dropped him off about half an hour before school. At the right time we sent him off to carefully cross the road at the designated crosswalk while we watched him. He had to be picked up by a pre-approved adult, so we arranged for Joe to walk across the playground to pick him up. My grandson, William, often came with them for a play time at Nanna's house. Mom and Dad were affectionately called "G&G" by the kids. Adan's dad often was finished work early for the day and would pick up Adan right from school.

At the foot of the stairs, at one end of Joe's living space, I organized a play area for the kids for after school. They never had more than an hour and a half before they were picked up by a parent. That was only when it was cold outside; otherwise they could play across the street in the playground if they stayed where we could see them. We could step out onto the front porch and call them back. It was so spiritually nourishing for Mom and Dad to have that much youthful activity around them for a short time each day. It was just enough to perk them up and not too much to wear them out.

Adan soon learned to ignore my mother's accusations and comments like, "You're a naughty boy!" said for no reason, or Dad telling him not to wear his hat in the house. The children were never there on weekends, so the house took on a different pace with whichever of us was on duty for the weekend. We each had our own space in the house, our own corners in which to find solace and be undisturbed. This was more "win-win" for all of us.

This added $900 into the piggy bank each month and took off some of the pressure for me to have the funds we needed and wanted without taking more from their nest egg. Since outings and life experiences are still helpful to those with dementia, it also gave us the resources to pay the fees for places and events, and the travel expenses.

At the year end, when taxes were due to be filed, I consulted with my accountant about declaring the income from the rental of the basement to Joe and the childcare for Adan. Because the rental was so far below the standard rate, we were advised not to claim it. However, because Adan's parents needed receipts from the childcare to write off on their taxes, we made those and claimed the income. It never amounted to enough to affect Mom and Dad's income tax.

Back to Work

Working with Parents in Tow

You can imagine my surprise when I took a phone call as I was driving Mom and Dad to an appointment downtown one day. I recognized the call as a contractor I had worked with doing leasehold improvements for former clients in retail. He said, "I have some clients that need your help. I looked all over the internet and can't find you anywhere! What happened?" I told him I had shut down the company to care for my parents full time. "Linda, would you consider just doing this one little job? They have an architect, but I need your way of communicating, like your sketches, color boards and samples boards to help them make decisions. Can I give them your contact information?"

I reluctantly said okay. When I met with them, I told them I came with two other people who might be along for the ride frequently. They said they didn't care. They were setting up a professional therapeutic massage center. I still recall the first time I took Mom in the transport chair with her coffee into the construction zone. She chatted with the trades and delighted them all by telling them how handsome they were! We both had drywall dust all over us when we left. Dad stayed in the car with his coffee and worked on one of his word search puzzles because I knew there would be no place dust free for him to sit.

A few more projects found their way into my life, but it was always on the condition that my parents care came first. Two times I had to leave a project during a meeting because I got a call from the nurse regarding Mom's episodes of not cooperating with her and Dad directing things with his cane which concerned the nurse. Even though the clients expressed disappointment at having to finish the meetings on the phone, online, or through emails, I never felt bad because they had hired me on that very clear condition.

Having their home as home base for my business ventures meant I could be in two places at the same time and deal with what was going on. Most of the time, just my presence in the house would calm things down. Dad would be stopped from "disciplining" Mom with his cane or saying mean things. Mom would be comforted and distracted or freshened up with a visit to the bathroom. The nurse did her best and I knew I didn't get an SOS call unless things were threatening to get out of her control. I also had my daughter just around the corner to call on if I couldn't get back in reasonable time.

I made a deal with one of my clients whose boutique fashion store I had helped to renovate. In exchange for a half day of merchandising and display, especially in the front windows, I was given beautiful, high fashion garments and accessories. This not only gave me an opportunity to keep my hand in the field of creative merchandising, but I always looked like the million dollars I didn't have! When clients commented on my outfits, I could always promote her and her store.

Mom came with me once, just to see how she would do, and as usual she wanted to go home to "Johnny" when she realized he wasn't there with us.

They settled into my working and the house became "home" even with "Linda's business" always somewhere in the space. Whether it was family, friends, or a client visiting, they always found our arrangement fascinating, interesting, and unusual for the norm.

It worked for us. That's what counted the most.

Done With Dementia

Linda McKendry

Routine Reigns
Routine Reigns

The one good thing about their stay at the Aspen Lodge was the routine they adopted and seemed to keep even when we moved them to the house in Haysboro. At the Aspen Lodge, breakfast could be skipped, and no one was concerned, or you could come down to breakfast in the dining room more at your leisure. You could also sit where you wanted, though lunch and dinner had assigned seating. This was because there were two sittings for the main meals due to the number of residents. You had to pick which sitting you preferred when you first arrived and then that was written in stone. There were days when Mom and Dad were out and about, visiting, shopping, or at appointments and would suddenly panic because they wouldn't make it in time for the meal. Dad was still driving, even after we moved them to Haysboro, and having the meals served right on the minute became extra important to him. To avoid stress, we made every effort to have meals ready at a specific time each day. This also made it easier for those helping to know what to plan and prepare for.

I didn't know if the habits they had at their old house would kick in now that they were back in their own home. It appears those seven months at the Lodge had spoiled Dad for going back to cooking their breakfast. We already knew Mom had stopped cooking before they moved into the Lodge. We were ready to pick up what needed to be done but do it the way they enjoyed before the lodge. We made their hot oatmeal just the way they liked it and added the dates, raisins, and flax after we put the plain version in Mom's bowl. The brown sugar and the milk or cream went on top of the half banana Dad cut up for his breakfast and automatically handed the other half to Mom. These were little things they had done for years.

Before they moved to the Aspen Lodge their routines were off. I would come by when they would normally be eating and find that they didn't have anything prepared, planned, or expected. Each of them would get busy with their own interests or would be out and about and not be worrying about meals. Dad was used to having Mom look after all that and Mom was now in more severe stages of dementia where making a meal didn't occur to her at all. This caused some conflict that would upset Mom, but she would still try. They laughed about Dad finding some eggs in his dresser drawer as he poked fun at Mom and teased her about how she was going to cook them in the drawer or did she just "lay them in there!" Ha! But again, these were signs that some routines were totally out of order or non-existent. I was visiting once when Dad came in with supper. Laughing he produced a large bag of donuts stating that they were just $1 at the grocery store because they were day old. Mom chided him and I asked, "Seriously. What are you guys having for supper?" Mom said, "I don't know," and Dad announced that they had the other half of a Meals on Wheels sandwich, bowl of soup, some crackers, and a little square for dessert. Once again, the other "half" was exactly the same thing delivered for two people two days before.

If it hadn't been for the meal routine at the Lodge they would have suffered even more. Once we had them in their own home, we saw immediately we had to construct some schedules and make routines that they and caregivers could follow. It was always easier to have a caregiver leave after preparing and serving a meal, then to be just coming when the meal needed to be prepared right away. If the dishes got left awhile it wasn't as critical as if the dinner was late getting served.

We also tried to fit appointments around the naps as much as possible. Naptime was always followed by good old English "teatime" and included a biscuit of some description. It also made the 8:00 pm snack time a leisurely evening with time for outings before getting ready for bed at 9:00. For Dad the highlight was his monthly clock club meeting. So, with Mom in tow, I would make sure we got him there for that and then picked him up. On those nights they were often in bed later than usual, but happy.

The daily 9-5 routine was also when the chores for the household were scheduled and fit in with the job description of the paid help. Our two foreign nurses didn't drive and wouldn't get their driver's licenses even though we offered to hire instructors. We had two vehicles available so one could have always been available for a nurse to take Mom and Dad to appointments, especially for hair dressing, foot care, and grocery shopping. I preferred to accompany them to medical appointments so I could stay informed. I tried to schedule these when I was on duty and the nurse would come along for support and to get any specific instructions for additional care. Because we had 24/7 care involving nurses, many of our medical professionals prescribed therapy or treatments we would have otherwise had to make separate appointments for.

We routinely used a single transport chair for both. Even though they were both mobile it was like having a park bench on the move. Either one could sit and rest in the chair being pushed by one of us while the other one walked. We took turns doing this so that we could navigate further and faster without so many stops for rest.

For exercise in the winter, I would drop them off at the far end of a mall with a food court and one of them would push the other and take turns while the nurse just walked along to keep an eye on them. Like having a walker, each could go further and faster, which was also the case if they were behind a shopping cart. It wasn't uncommon to see the two of them walking side by side behind a shopping cart with their canes sticking out of it and people smiling at them as they passed by. This made all our routine shopping and exercise excursions safer and time saving.

Bedtime routine was always helping Mom more than Dad except when he first came home from the hospital and was recovering from his crisis. Dad would never be seen outside the bedroom without being fully dressed. Mom on the other hand was comfortable in her nightgown and housecoat any time of the day and would often come to breakfast dressed this way. This was the best way to have them sitting down at the same time to eat without making Dad wait while we helped Mom.

We brought the dressers from their original home and Dad was in and out of his daily while he did his dressing and grooming. His laundry basket filled as he regularly changed his shirt, pants, and underwear. We also gave him the same side of the double closet that he had in their home for years. Mom on the other hand, was content to stay in her nightgown and housecoat until someone said, "Come, Mom. Let's get dressed." And then she would get up and follow you into the bedroom or bathroom. She would let you pick her clothes and like dressing a small child, you would have to give instruction at every step, but she would help by putting her arm in a sleeve or lifting her foot to go into a pant leg. She would also button up her own blouses. She had stopped wearing bras because they cut into her shoulders where she had lost the use of the ligaments. We substituted nice soft undershirts which she wore day and night. She wore cozy flannel nightgowns, a fleecy housecoat, and closed toe slippers with leather soles and socks.

Linda McKendry

A little trick we all used when helping her dress for bed in the winter was to lay her night clothes on the heat vent in the bathroom. She would often comment on how nice they felt.

It occurred to me that each time she looked up at the closet, she would just put on what she saw first without thinking, then do it again and again. It was also obvious that Dad wasn't of the mind to get up and take her in, or help her, as he would have at least remembered it was a sweater she needed.

He was fiercely independent and so much a gentleman who refused to wear sweatpants one day more than he had to after his abdominal surgery. I purchased dress pants many sizes larger than he really needed, to wear with suspenders, and be comfortable with an ileostomy bag that needed room to expand especially when he sat down. He had never worn jeans in his whole life and was proud of that. Jeans were for farm work and he had to wear them as a boy. Somewhere he had made up his mind that when he was old enough to choose his own clothes, they would be dressier. Even in India, in each picture he is wearing khaki pants and a seer sucker shirt, always looking "dapper" and well dressed.

These were the things that were important to take care of in their routines. Included in them was the schedule for prescription medications, exercises, and for Dad going out as often as he could get someone to take him. On warmer days he and Mom would often go for a little walk down the block to the end and back, but I put a stop to that the day I saw Dad using his cane to steer Mom where he wanted to turn. It wasn't a gentle tap. After that I would just get them into the car and drive them to a coffee shop or drive through to pick up a coffee and go sit in a park. Not much exercise, but at least keeping Mom safe from "cane correcting."

Routines also kept them looking forward to the next event in the day and more than that, helping the caregivers know what to do and when to do it. It made their lives more consistent with different caregivers coming and going. Weekends were a little more flexible and lunch was often on the way home from church, if the nap wasn't delayed too much. It also made for a day that was peaceful and pleasant for all involved.

I knew that in a nursing home, firstly they wouldn't be together, and secondly there would be activities and noise from televisions and music that they didn't like or enjoy. This way we could make a life for them daily that was full of what they liked the most in the place they called home. I knew there were routines and schedules in the facilities to accommodate all the residents and staff, and in some cases not as flexible, or personal, as ours, but I also knew that only having two residents to worry about made it a lot easier.

Two Birds and One Stone

Two Birds and One Stone

One of the reasons facilities for groups of people work is because you don't need the one on one care all the time. It's just as easy to cook for two or three as it is for one, mostly because of the food package sizes. It didn't cost any more for rent, utilities, or outings in the car when more than one person was being covered. When Joe came to stay with us as a border, our rent didn't go up and our utilities only went up a tiny bit. I increased the grocery budget a little. But we kept the same menus and meal planning process which became routine. The rule was to only plan leftovers if there was enough for a complete meal the next day for all three of them.

Funding Combined

The Self Managed Care Funding was recommended to me by the Home Care Nurse supervisor. She called to let me know there was a training session at one of the hospitals. There was only room for 100 and there were two spots left. She felt I would be a good candidate to manage funding for hiring care for Mom and Dad. It was a two-hour session and we were handed large three-inch blue binders with tabs and pages and pages of information. It was made clear that there was funding available but there were a lot of conditions for the use of it and reports had to be made every six months. We already had our nurse in place, and we were paying her the minimum required by immigration and subsidizing it.

I felt overwhelmed by the information and process, but I also recognized the potential and decided I would be willing to give it a try. Running my own consulting business for eighteen years gave me a good comprehension of the use of accounting software into which I could download tax and employee deduction charts.

I could generate reports to make the reconciling easier and I was already doing online banking for Mom and Dad. I signed up to be put on the waiting list. The supervisor made an appointment to come and assess our needs, which she said would determine the funds we would get. She went on to explain that each of them would be assessed separately based on their individual needs, but I could pool the funds to use to hire one person to look after both at the same time.

While we were carrying on waiting for approval for the funding, Dad had his surgery and collapsed from septic shock four days later. Because he was in the hospital and not being cared for at home the funding would not come at that time. The funding for Mom kicked in while Dad was in the hospital. However, much to my surprise, the supervisor came over to tell me that they had special emergency funding that Dad qualified for and because his needs increased when he came home to recover, the funds increased from the original assessment. The funds were deposited automatically in their bank accounts and I evened out the amounts each month so that each of them paid our nurse, and any other paid help, exactly 50% each. This was because I had to set each of them up as a formal business with a tax number and deal with holiday pay, income tax deductions, pensions, and unemployment insurance.

The nurses were paid every two weeks while others were paid each day they worked. This funding reduced the amount we had to subsidize so more was staying in Mom and Dad's investment to generate a little more interest. It also provided the overall care, light housekeeping, meal preparation and monitoring medical prescriptions for three people, including what Joe needed.

So many times, we only needed one person to keep an eye on both of them at the same time. I knew that if either of them became immobile, bedridden, or suffered some other condition, that might change, but most of the time one person could be there for all of them. The main issue was the nurses who Mom would not cooperate with. This meant that we had to leave clear instruction on how to get Dad to convince Mom to do what was necessary. It also meant that sometimes she wouldn't get fresh underwear right after a little accident. But the pull-ups were made of material that kept moisture away from the skin for many hours with no leaking or odor. Mom would never change herself, but she would try to wipe off the underwear, putting the soiled toilet paper into the garbage can. Since we had a routine for taking care of that, it was never a problem.

The Self Managed Care Funding was regulated so that it could not be used to pay immediate family for their care. We also couldn't use the same agencies that Home Care used. A small contingency in the Fund could be used to advertise for help. We found out that it was easier to have a full time foreign nurse, and later a Canadian student nurse, then to piecemeal each need we had to different people at different times. One to come for meal preparation. One to come for light housekeeping and laundry. One to come for respite care. One to come for companionship. That would have been a nightmare for me to organize and pay. For people with dementia it would also have been confusing.

The Caregiver's Room

The bedroom set up for family and overnight caregivers was also organized so anyone could use it and be comfortable. The best thing about the room is that it was adjacent to the bathroom and with the door open a crack you could watch for Mom or Dad getting up in the night. A beautiful angel night light in the hall gave enough light to use the bathroom without turning on the main light if the bathroom door was kept open. With their bedroom on the other side we could hear them talking, making a fuss about something, or in some cases Mom spitting or throwing up. This one room was used by all who came. It also had a wall mounted TV. Once Mom and Dad were asleep, very little would disturb them.

Each person who came had to learn how to empty Dad's bag at his request, and never let it go more than five hours. Mom never commented on this condition and learned to wait for Dad to come back from his "bunk" while she watched TV or her favorite gospel musical videos. If she did wander around to find where he had gone, she would just hover outside the door to the room because he had shooed her away so many times.

The only time they could be separated for a short period of time was if one of us took Mom somewhere and left Dad with a nurse. Otherwise we had to take both. When I say "we" I mean one of us kids, or someone they knew well. And whoever was there had to use a parenting "authoritative" voice, which the nurses never did. They were hard workers and very diligent, but soft spoken and too shy to speak with authority to either Mom or Dad.

Linda McKendry

Program Waiting Lists

There were many programs available for seniors and all of them were based on the individual. So when I put their names on the waiting list often only one name would come up. If it was Dad's name, he could go on his own and that wouldn't be a problem. If it was Mom's name then one of us had to be there, or Dad had to be there. One program recognized our situation and they arranged for Mom to come as Dad's "companion" when they saw how much fun she had being with Dad in the social setting. However, there were issues and Dad's idea of correcting Mom was seen as a form of verbal abuse and bullying, so we were asked to keep her home. We were just happy that the program organizers had tried and made an exception so they could stay together.

The whole system was based on the individual and when I looked around for a facility that could care for them the way we were nothing stacked up as good. The logistics didn't work because of the facility layout and design didn't accommodate them as a couple. We would have to show up or pay someone to bring them together as much as possible which would never include sleeping together, or even in the same room, except for meals. The cost was also two to three times what we were spending each month. We did visit one facility where they were in the process of building a floor that would keep couples together regardless of the difference in medical and mental conditions. It was three years away and already had a waiting list. I sometimes feel like going by and checking it out all these years later.

All the caregivers, family, friends, and nurses loved to come and be there for us. Whether they got paid or not they knew that any chore, job, task, or assignment (favor) was designed to look after both at the same time with the least amount of trouble or stress. The multi-function of so many spaces made it easier for each person to be safe, sound and sane.

Building the Team

Me first. Every team needs a leader and someone to build a team. I was that person who had accepted the responsibility and had the legal authority to make decisions on our parents' behalf. I hadn't solidified the help and I had done as much as I could by myself. As I thought of this chapter, because I couldn't have done what we did alone as it turned out, I realized that the next members of the team were Mom and Dad themselves.

We needed Dad to help us direct Mom since she would always listen to him and try to do what he said. We had to make sure he wasn't being abusive or mean, but it was so helpful to know Dad could be counted to give Mom direction. This was particularly helpful to the foreign nurses when Mom wouldn't respect them or listen to them. However, Dad would often rebuke her for telling the nurses they were stupid, and it felt like no one was happy. Most of Dad's contribution to our team was just being within sight and sound of Mom since she lived to know where he was.

Mom was part of the team because Dad needed her too. She was constantly telling him how wonderful he was and still laughing at his jokes. It was obvious to us sometimes that she didn't understand or remember the joke, but she seemed to know intuitively or by habit when to laugh and we knew that made him feel good. She was still comforting to him and would do everything she could to make him happy. We knew that they were still having "hugs and cuddles" in their private bedroom time. We were careful never to interfere when we could hear them having intimate conversations.

The next people on the team, most of whom had already been there but not servicing daily needs, were the medical professionals, including the pharmacist they had for years. Visiting many of the doctors, technicians, dentists, foot and hair care people always felt like a social event. This is one of the reasons I went out of my way to make sure they had the same contacts they were familiar with.

Closer to home the team member I made the first important decisions with was my sister, Susie. She ended every conversation with, "Call if you need anything." And I knew she meant it. I had witnessed her care for Mom and Dad over the years and knew of her desire to have Mom and Dad live with them as I've already stated. She and I were free to consult with her husband Terry to get medical clarification or help with treating minor symptoms. That was invaluable.

Next on my list were the live-in nurses, Sol and Josie, who we hired with the funding provided. At one point we did have two on minimum wage based on an agreement when they needed the work and cash flow, but we didn't know at the time which one was going to be with us permanently. Sol lived in, and Josie came on duty from the apartment she shared with other friends from her country. The third, Erin, was a Canadian student nurse who was there when Mom and Dad passed away and hired to help Dad when he went into the veteran's home.

The best part of the team was my siblings and their spouses. This was great for me because I knew I could trust them to take care of Mom and Dad in a way they enjoyed. It also gave Mom and Dad that extra familiar element each month. My siblings came on scheduled weekends so I could have quality time off and avoid paying a nurse overtime on statutory holidays. They were there at our family meetings to help make decisions concerning the overall

Linda McKendry

care. I turned to my brother Gary to help me with the budgeting and arranging of the cash flow subsidies from their nest egg. The boys were also the handymen we needed from time to time to install, fix, or retrofit a fixture to fit their space.

On the fringe were other trusted family members and friends, who I felt free to call on to contribute to special needs from time to time. Some were scheduled and some spontaneous. The most important was my daughter Kim. She lived so close and was my first emergency call if it wasn't 911. Often, we had four generations for lunch or after school snacks when her children were there. It was win-win as each generation got to know the other one better. It created a greater appreciation for having family close by for help or for fun.

I can include the landlords, neighbors, our senior boarder, Joe, and our after school care student, Adan and his parents. It was a big team. My main job was to communicate with them, so every day's schedule was covered one way or another.

First Responders

When you are caregiving anyone who is not safe to be left alone, whether a small child, a disabled person, or people who are frail in body and weak in mind, whoever is on duty as the primary caregiver is a first responder.

Even when we teach a teenager to care for little kids so they can earn money babysitting, we teach them what to do in case of emergency. Before that we must constitute what determines an emergency. If the child is crying because the parent is leaving for the evening, that isn't an emergency, except to the child. In the same way when we were caring for Mom and Dad, we had to determine what constituted an emergency that would result in a call to 911.

This is where family came in as our "first responders" who we solicited to step in and help. Why family first?

- They usually know more about the loved one than others.
- They are perceived to have a moral duty and conscience towards caring for another family member.
- They are often living in close proximity relatively speaking.
- They can often at least contribute in tangible ways if they can't personally be there.
- They are usually willing to or obligated to volunteer and put in their time without expecting to be paid.
- They might be in the will and thus willing to "pay it forward" as they say.
- They usually get the information and respect they need on behalf of the loved one when they identify themselves as "family."

Linda McKendry

There can be a difference between the family member who has the greatest desire to help but also has the least ability or sensibility. Experience dealing with people, communicating, and other factors play into getting the right kind of help. Having said this though there are always places where someone willing to help can find something to do. In any case there needs to be a good backup.

When I was gone from the house and the nurses were on duty, I knew that I had to have a backup for Mom in case she had an episode. This was Kim, my daughter who, as I've said, lived a couple of blocks away and was at that time a full-time stay-at-home mother. As long as the nurse could keep Mom in the confines of the house or a room and coach Dad on how to help her without using his cane, things were manageable until Kim could get there. Kim talks about the times when she would have to use her "mother" voice and call her grandma "Lydia," using her first name to get her attention and a positive response.

Wherever there was any doubt about the caregiver's abilities, I would have back up. There were very few episodes on weekends when the nurse was off duty completely. But when the nurse was a live in, she could be called to come up and take blood pressure or give a professional medical opinion to determine if something was an emergency or not.

When Dad had his first seizure, he was eating his oatmeal at breakfast. I saw his eyes roll back and his head begin to fall forward. I quickly pulled away his bowl so his face wouldn't fall into it. He passed out and began to lean precariously to the side of the armchair that I imagined would tip over if he kept going that way. I held him up and hollered for the nurse who came quickly.

Between the two of us, we laid him down on the floor and she ran to get the blood pressure machine while I ran to get a little pillow for under his head.

While the nurse worked on him and listened to his heart with the stethoscope, I checked on Mom who was continuing to eat her oatmeal as if nothing had happened. I knew she was fine. I got my cell phone and called 911.

We were close to a hospital, so an ambulance was there in about five minutes. Dad opened his eyes and looked around at the EMS people and at the wires they were attaching to him for the ECG machine. They reassured him he was going to be okay. He looked over at me and I just said, "Dad you passed out at the table, so we called the ambulance. You're in good hands now." They determined his oxygen level was low, but his heart was strong, lungs sounded good, so it was time to decide if he should go to the hospital or not. The EMS people said that we could call them to come back if necessary. Fortunately with our Canadian Health Care system there would be no charge for ambulance service. We also checked his blood sugar because he was diabetic, and it was normal. He had eaten half his oatmeal and said he was still hungry.

We decided that was a good sign to just leave him home for now and the EMS people left after tearing off the ECG report, which I put in the file in the pocket on the side of the fridge for later reference if I needed it.

A few days later he collapsed again. My memory isn't serving me accurately about all the details, such as, how many, what time, when or where. I do know that he was hospitalized one of those times and they couldn't find any reason for it and on the chart they wrote: "Old Age - 89 years old!"

Each time he was in the hospital and ready to be discharged the Alberta Health Care people would come and find out what his living arrangements were so they could advise where to send him. Many seniors are delivered to the emergency from the home they are still living in, but don't always go back there due to the system. I was always happy to tell them we had the Self Managed Care Funding, a live-in nurse, and around the clock care.

If either of them were in a full care facility, like a hospital, for more than ten days, then the rule was that the funding was stopped until at least two weeks being home and assessed as "stable" by a home care supervisor. We found out that usually meant that the funding was increased because there would often be increased needs for hired care after a hospital stay or crisis. We didn't want to lose our funding because we depended on it to subsidize the "nest egg" we were taking from on a regular basis. I had everything budgeted tight, but we didn't lack.

Mom would have TIAs (Transient Ischemic Attack) caused by a temporary clot from time to time and we knew the symptoms for these. We also knew that taking her to the hospital or calling 911 would result in an unnecessary trip. We were told that older people have these and don't equate symptoms like tiredness or weakness in a limb with a stroke. For Mom, our first clue was that by nine in the morning she still hadn't gotten up for breakfast. Then there might be a little struggle to get her spoon to her mouth. On a couple of occasions, she walked for a few hours with a little drag in one leg. These would go away and she would recover to what was her "normal" so we didn't do anything about it. We knew that if you know or suspect someone is having a stroke, you

Done With Dementia

have them take an 81mg aspirin and get to the hospital as soon as possible to prevent or lessen damage due to a clot. In Mom's case she wasn't able to tell us this so by the time we noticed a symptom, usually many hours later, we would know what it was. We just helped her along and kept an eye on her and let her sleep as long as she wanted to.

Dad on the other hand had a DVT (blood clot in the vein) in his leg. He didn't say anything, and I didn't pick up on it. My brother-in-law doctor happened to be staying over on one of their weekends and suspected it so he took Dad into emergency to have it checked out. That was when he was put on Warfarin and we had to take him regularly to have his blood tested and the INR reported so we knew what dosage to give him and when to come in for the next test.

I can't remember if it was the same occasion, but I remember taking them to church and someone came up to me after and asked if Dad had suffered a stroke because of the way in which his arm was kind of dangling by his side. I do remember our appointment at the hospital stroke clinic for home care instructions including diet and symptoms to watch for. The little consult room was full with me, Dad, Mom, and our nurse. The doctor was filling out a form and asking Dad a lot of questions. She didn't look up as she asked the next question. "Do you bruise easily?" And he answered, "Only when they hit me with the rolling pin." I saw her writing down what he was saying and then she looked up to see us all shaking our heads and laughing because Dad was such a joker.

This joking also reminds me of a pre-op exam Dad had for his lungs. He was asked if he had ever smoked. He replied, "Oh, just a little cigar once in a while!" I was shocked at his answer and immediately corrected this. Dad had never touched alcohol or

161

tobacco in his life because of his strict upbringing. We all knew the consequences in our family if we were ever caught smoking. I chided him and he just chuckled at having some fun with the doctor. Thank God I was there with him. And this was the story of taking care of them. Someone had to be there to give the correct answers because either they couldn't remember, the memory was false, or Dad was just joking.

Emergency Away from Home

We took Mom and Dad up to Susie's for a little holiday while we parked our holiday trailer at a campground nearby. Mom hadn't been feeling well and had a terrible cough. She was resisting fluids, not cooperating in taking her prescription medications, generally suffering and in a bad mood. Nothing we did was cheering her up and she was most content just dozing on Susie's couch in the living room. Even at the table she wasn't eating much. Terry arranged to take her to his hospital and had a chest x-ray done. As he studied it with one of his colleagues, they noticed a little spot in the lung that was symptomatic of something serious. They prescribed a very strong, specific antibiotic, but in the next few days she became more lethargic and struggled to take the medication or drink anything. We called the brothers and told them we weren't sure if Mom was going to have a turn around or not. They were alerted to be ready to drive up if she continued to get worse.

Having a doctor as a First Responder is always great comfort. Susie drove all the way to the campground to give us the news because we were out of cell phone range. I was concerned about Mom but not worried. I continued to enjoy our little time away knowing that Mom was in the best hands possible. My sister is the proverbial pampering person and had a special relationship with Mom, but even she was becoming a little frustrated that none of the tactics she usually used to get Mom to eat or drink were working.

All of us who cared for Mom and Dad were the First Responders. We were there when anything extreme or out of the ordinary happened to make the decision to call 911 or just deal with it in the moment and do a little "wait and see." Having the nurse there to take blood pressure and check pulse was comforting as well. Some things that were an emergency the first time weren't after that when we knew the cause and usual outcome. Also, dealing with people of "old age" we knew we had the option of just letting them go peacefully and in the comfort of palliative care. If Mom had not begun to eat again, we would have had harder choices to make. We always told the EMS and doctors: "We are a family of faith. We hope for the best, but we are prepared for the worst." That brought comfort to them too, doing their best to treat our parents.

We made Mom as comfortable as possible for the eight-hour drive back to Calgary with the idea that she needed to see their gerontologist and be closer to the medical team and facilities in Calgary. From where Susie and Terry lived it was a helicopter ride to the nearest hospital capable of extended care. I called Dr. Cohen when we got into Calgary and was told what the options were even before we got an appointment. She said that if we couldn't get Mom to eat we had the option of a feeding tube. With all the resistance we had just taking her blood pressure, I knew a feeding tube would be a real challenge. The other option was to just monitor her and if she got really weak, frail, and was fading, we would consider administering palliative care for comfort.

While waiting to take Mom to her appointment with Dr. Cohen, I thought of Mom's all-time favorite food. Lemon meringue pie. I went to the store immediately and bought one. We offered her a piece and she ate it. Not the crust, mind you. But I looked at that and thought, "We have lemon with some vitamin C, and we have egg white with a little protein." This was eaten with a few sips of tea that had milk in it. I told the nurse, "I don't care if you have to give her lemon pie for breakfast, lunch, dinner, and every snack, if she's eating it then do it." That evening the nurse served a half a rack of mini ribs done in the oven with BBQ sauce. Dad thought he was going to have this feast all to himself until Mom reached over and took one off his plate. I rescued her hand from his fork when he objected by reminding him that we were trying to get her to eat. She ended up having three of them. Dad was grumpy.

I was elated. That seemed to kick-start her appetite and obviously her body was recovering, and she was feeling better overall.

By the time we got to Dr. Cohen's Mom was back to her old self and telling Dr. Cohen she was "still alive and kicking," as she lifted her foot to give a little kick in the air. Dr. Cohen looked at me as if to ask if I had been lying or exaggerating when I called earlier. I told her about the lemon pie and the ribs. I didn't have to decide between a feeding tube and palliative care. Thank God.

Friends Second

Mom and Dad had friends they knew and trusted. I knew that I could call on any one of them and they were likely to do what they could to help. One of them, a neighbor across the street from their original home, had cared for her husband many years and he had died in her arms when his end came. She had moved into an apartment close to where they now lived. They loved her so I approached her to drive them around and stay with them at the house making tea and entertaining them until one of us arrived to take over. I trusted her completely because of the emergencies she had dealt with looking after her husband. Everyone had my cell number and other contact numbers were listed on the bulletin board in the kitchen.

I hired the daughter of friends of Mom and Dad's, along with her fiancé, to come on Sunday mornings to pick up Mom and Dad and take them to church. I gave them some cash to cover the cost of Sunday lunch before bringing them home. Then they stayed with them during their afternoon nap. Her mother has recently passed away after a very long bout with malignant tumors and I knew that she had some experience with emergencies and serious medical issues. Not only did this give me confidence to leave Mom and Dad in their care. This gave me the respite I needed, to spend more time in my own home with my husband on Sunday.

Others When You Need Them:

Once when Dad was having one seizure after another, I called 911 and he was taken to the hospital. There are four hospitals in Calgary. I couldn't go with them or meet up with him until I had care for Mom. They said they were taking him to the Peter Lougheed Hospital, but when I drove over there, I found out they had re-routed them to the Foothills which was completely the other side of the city. When I finally got there, Dad was still having the seizures. It became common to watch. I wasn't even reacting anymore. After all he was in emergency at a hospital and they were responsible. At one point a nurse came in and asked if he had been seen by the doctor yet. I gave her my saga of tracking him down saying I had just arrived a few minutes ago. She watched over my shoulder as he had another seizure. She went over to him to feel the pulse in his wrist and asked me how long this had been going on. I told her since I had called the EMS at home several hours ago.

For some reason that put her into high gear and she immediately got the doctor to come and examine him. In the end he was tested and given a medication to stop the seizures and sent home with the referral to a specialist. The specialist did more testing and put him on a medication he was on the rest of his life with no more seizures or significant side effects.

There were two times when I drove them to the emergency room at nearby hospitals and because the wait times were getting longer and longer, I eventually just took them home. I remember thinking that if they had passed that length of time with nothing getting worse; I would deal with it on my own. I did have Doctor Google, after all, to check symptoms for severity, DIY treatments, and advice for what to watch for if it got worse. I also had Dr. Unger, my sister's husband who was a GP in a remote hospital. Every time we had any procedures or tests done; we would put his name on the chart to be notified of the results. That way we could also consult with him, especially to explain in laymen's terms what we were dealing with, even when he couldn't give treatment.

All the diagnosis was coming down to what happens when we age. With Mom and Dad in their early 90s at this point, we knew it was just a matter of time before something about "old age" would do them in for good. It would be an emergency we couldn't do anything about.

Making Everything Work

This chapter provides a methodical list of what we did to create flow from one space to another, and from one shift to another. Planning and preparing for meals, household chores, laundry and everyday care made the entire process more enjoyable. Each time I pushed the button for Main in an elevator while caring for Mom and Dad, I would think of all the "Ms" I had to have in place. I decided to make a list of them to share how we created a flow that kept things moving forward the best way possible. They became known as my M&Ms.

Follow the "M&Ms" to determine some of the ways to prevent burnout and facilitate sharing responsibilities.

MANAGE

- <u>SCHEDULES</u>: The more people you have as caregivers, the more important it is to post a calendar, a bulletin board, and a white board for daily reminders. In our case the wall space behind the back door in the kitchen was the place I chose. It was central and everyone spent time in the kitchen no matter what.

We had internet installed in the house so that we could send emails, reports, and other information electronically, but the good old-fashioned wall calendar and bulletin board were still vital. In addition to this I also had their medical records in a magnetic file pocket attached to the side of the fridge, and a journal/log book that went with the medications for when we were giving temporary meds due to an injury or special condition. Each had a special place and everyone knew where to look for the information they wanted or needed.

Linda McKendry

- Master Calendar
- Appointments
- Caregivers' Schedule
- Leisure Activities & Events

Example: Master Calendar 2010

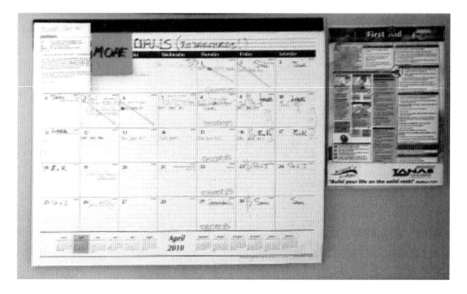

This is what our master calendar looked like. It was large enough to write things on. In 2010 we were already in the monthly rotation of each sibling coming and taking one weekend from Friday evening at five when the nurse went off duty to Monday morning at nine when she came back. During the week, I came on duty at five and stayed the night. You can see that next to it is a one page First Aid Chart I felt would be useful for those of us not trained as nurses.

Done With Dementia

Example: Master Calendar 2013

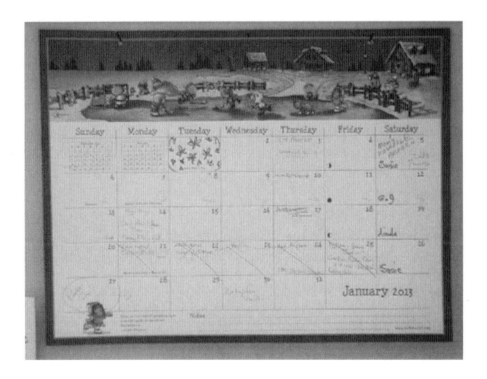

Mom passed away on December 21, 2012. The day all the ancient calendars ended! This calendar was already filled in for each week with events, appointments, and caregivers we were expecting.

All the stars are for New Year's Day and there's a note on Saturday the 5th for Mom's burial and memorial service. Another note shows Dad going to the farm where my brother Gary lived and all the appointments listed in the third week were crossed off. Life changed from then on.

Linda McKendry

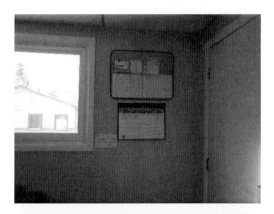

- Master Bulletin Board – contacts and communication
- Daily Routine
- Important Contacts
- EMS
- Notices
- Reminders
- <u>Daily Routine</u>: This list was just a reminder for those who came regularly and a quick review for those who just tucked in occasionally to help out.

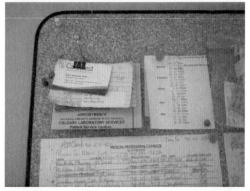

- <u>Contact List</u>: Most of the time I was the one taking them to their appointments and most of these contacts were in my cell phone. But for those who were on duty, and especially if there was an emergency, I wanted everyone to have the important numbers.

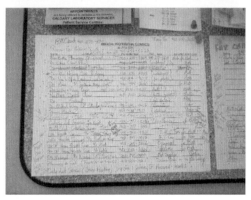

These could be stored in cell phones too.

The list got longer as we had more people helping and more appointments with specialists. It got a little messy as some were changed or crossed off. I felt it was more important to keep it current than worry about how pretty it looked. My time was valuable.

NOTE: If you are reading this as an eBook, you can zoom in and see how I made the list. I noted if the contact was just for Mom, or Dad, or for both. They both had the same eye doctor, hearing aid specialist, general physician, bowel surgeon, gerontologist, pedicurist, and pharmacist. They had different hair stylists, and each had some medical issues that were seen by specialists. Dad's were for his diabetes, heart and lungs, seizures, DVT, and of course, the clinics for his ileostomy care.

- Mini White Board: We kept a mini white board on the top of the microwave. On this we put the day of the week, the month, and the year. We then put a notice, reminder, or 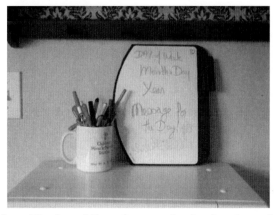 a cute saying for the day. Dad and Joe always looked at it and read it. Mom didn't even know it was there.

I can recall the number of times Mom was assessed for her medication and part of the test was to ask her what season of the year it was. She would always say fall no matter what. I would coach her on the way to the doctor's if it was spring or summer... but she would still say "fall."

Linda McKendry

Mom and Dad were case studies at the University and their bowel surgeon and gerontologist were on the faculty. One day Dr. Cohen, the gerontologist, called to find out if two of her interns could come by and interview Mom and Dad. We said yes, knowing Mom and Dad would enjoy the attention and loved to have company.

You can imagine how much I laughed when they asked Mom what season of the year it was, and she said, "fall" which it was. I knew they were duly impressed, and she got four points for that answer! I explained the situation so they wouldn't be reporting wrong findings.

- SPACE: Use what you know about your parents' preferences to set up the space to suit their needs.

Each time we had to move or change things up, I measured the space. In each case I made a little floor plan to scale, measured up their furnishings and plotted them onto the plan making sure they would fit and the space around them would be adequate and safe.

This gave me a list of what to get rid of and what to keep and move. Keep in mind what is most familiar to them and what they prefer.

- Living Room: the chairs they sit in all the time are the most important piece of furniture you can keep. In some cases, you may have to upgrade to something safer, more ergonomic, or even a chair that electronically helps your parent get up and down safely. If you have to make a change, I suggest you either purchase one in the color to match what you are replacing or ask your parent if they see something they would like, assuming they can and want to make a choice.

- <u>Tables and Lamps</u>: Most people need a place to put their books, reading glasses, or beverage under adequate lighting. I recommend a good lamp with a pull chain and a good fob at the end. I also suggest the use of incandescent tri-light bulbs so the lighting can be adjusted to the function. Less light is needed for watching TV than for reading or doing puzzles. Some seniors use laptops and cell phones, so they need less light for those too.

After that the most important things to keep in the living room are some of the familiar photos, wall décor, and ornaments. A coffee table is okay if there's room and it won't be a tripping hazard.

- <u>Personal Belongings</u>: Each person who lived there and ongoing regular caregivers needed a place for personal belongings. This included the nurses who needed a secure place for their purses and backpacks. We let them store their personal things in the closet in the third bedroom.

Things like luggage, Dad's fishing gear, and off-season coats and footwear were kept in the back entrance closet. There was also a nice storage area down under the stairs and I put the Christmas decorations there, with party supplies and gift wrapping stuff. The children who came for after school care had their own little cubbies in shelf units, or boxes with their names on them in which to keep things they used a lot and wanted separate.

Joe, our boarder, had all his personal things downstairs in his suite. Our one live-in nurse had her own room and kept her personal things in it. We arranged to have a lock set put on the door of her bedroom so she would feel safe and secure. She and Joe shared the washroom and the kitchen which they organized to suit their needs.

- <u>Leisure and Entertainment Items</u>: Mom and Dad had a large collection of videos and DVDs of their favorite movies and Gospel music. We kept them in a special shelf unit under the TV in the darkest corner of the living room with the least amount of glare.

Dad had a little shelf unit against the wall where his chair was and it was loaded with all his puzzles, his dexterity balls, putty, and other things he used to exercise his hands. He had mugs with pens, scissors, tape... it was just a "junk" place to keep his personal entertainment items close by, in comfortable reach, and visible. A magazine rack was behind the table between him and Mom where he kept his stock of Word Search Puzzle books.

Mom had lost interest in things she had once done. Even though we had another magazine rack close to her with knitting and needle work kits in various stages of completion, she didn't notice them or even attempt any. We would often take one out and hand it to her. She might try, but it was lost as she couldn't figure out what to do.

One day I decided to cast on a few stitches for a knitting project she could work on. I handed it to her and she said, "What's this?" I said, "It's just something for you to do." "Well, what is it?" I again replied, "Well it can be whatever you want it to be. Maybe a scarf? Or a doll blanket?" "That's silly!" And she handed it back to me. Later I noticed she had picked it up and taken all the stitches off the needle without winding the yarn back on the ball. I didn't try again, but we left it there anyways.

- <u>Bedroom</u>: It didn't take long for me to realize that the old bed Mom and Dad had was becoming difficult for them to get in and out of. I did a shopping trip to a furniture store and found a beautiful white wrought- iron bed that had a headboard and foot board. It was quite high, so I purchased the high bedside tables as well. When we assembled and installed it, Mom and Dad tried it out and it was too high. They both felt like they would fall out and their feet didn't touch the floor when they sat on the sides.

My husband brought the hack saw and took a good six inches off each leg, which made it just the right height. The next purchase was a hospital grade antibacterial, waterproof mattress cover.

We also had to purchase new bedding to fit the bed and then equip it with their electric blanket which was under the mattress cover. It was turned on a few minutes before they went to bed and then set to go off automatically a few minutes after. This was something they had always done, and I knew that getting into a warm bed was a real comfort for both. Neither of them suffered from arthritis but Dad had a little joint pain in his hip.

The bedside lamps were the ones I had purchased for them years earlier which were tri-light touch lamps. Mom and Dad both knew to just reach over and touch the lamps to turn them off or on. As each of us had to get up in the middle of the night to empty Dad's bag, it was easy to touch the lamp for a very soft light and then touch it twice quickly to turn it off. The footboard on the bed was sturdy enough for either of them to hold onto as they went around it.

- Dining: Armchairs are important in any eating area too. Do not use chairs that have castors, even though they are easier to move. They are too unstable. The best chairs we ever got were from a nursing home being upgraded. What appeared to be a tweed fabric was actually a good grade of textured vinyl, making them easy to clean from spills or incontinence.

The table needs to be high enough for comfortable eating and for chair arms to fit under. Also, if your parent gets up by using the edge of the table for support and pushes the chair back with their legs, the table should be on rubber coasters so it won't slide.

- Grooming/Bathroom: I did everything I knew to do to keep the medicine cabinet the same as they had in their own house: Dad's toiletries to the far-left side and Mom's to the far-right. This was their toothbrushes, paste, hair care products, and denture rinses.

For Mom the most important supplies were her pull ups (never called diapers), the wipes, Kleenex, and the Glaxo Based cream we used for her when we helped her. The brand of pull ups she used fit beautifully and were leak-proof and odor-proof. A small lidded waste can within comfortable reach of the toilet was for her care also.

She could always hold her bladder when we were on the road, just announcing she needed a potty so we would stop in at the next service station or restaurant. I never apologized for using the washroom of a restaurant we didn't eat in. I would ask the waiters if they wanted anything for using it, just to be polite. They all seemed to understand, and it was always okay.

Because we went through so much Kleenex and recycled plastic grocery bags, I purchased a little cupboard/ drawer unit to place just outside the bathroom door to have for these items. The space under the sink of this mid-century house had sliding doors which I removed. I painted the inside a clean, white enamel and put extra towels on the open shelves on one side and stacks of Mom's pull ups on the toilet side.

Because of her dementia, she never thought to change her pull ups on her own. She would just wipe them and put the wipe in the lidded waste can. But they were in comfortable reach from the toilet so helping her was quick and easy for the rest of us.

Other:

- Dad's "Bunk": The main bedroom was for Mom and Dad and was set up as much like their original one as possible. The second bedroom next to the washroom and on the other side of the wall from Mom and Dad's room I set up as a caregiver's room. It had the wall mounted TV, an open shelf closet, a retro style dresser and chest of drawers. I assigned drawers and spaces to each of the siblings who came to stay overnight on weekends so they could keep stuff there and not have to pack and unpack each time.

The third bedroom had Dad's watch repair bench in one corner. Along the adjacent wall we put the hospital bed that had all the different adjustments, including controls to raise and lower it. This was used to change Dad's bag weekly and empty it several times daily. Dad called it "the Bunk". It was so handy for all of us to use since it removed the need to stoop by putting his body at the perfect height for nursing. I kept all the supplies in a tall shelf unit with drawers that I managed to get into one end of the closet. The hospital table displayed the ileostomy cleaning and changing supplies.

This table came in handy when we had to use it to block the hall so Mom wouldn't wander the wrong way when she came back from

Linda McKendry

using the bathroom a few times at night. We kept figuring out these things whenever we had an issue.

MAINTENANCE

- <u>Property Maintenance</u>: If your parents are still in their own home and need help in the house or around the yard this may be something you can fit into your normal schedule. Check with neighbors who are willing to whip over and give your parents' lawn a once over while they are doing their own. Offer to pay them a little or give them a gift card for a favorite store or eatery. This works for removing snow too.

Housekeeping depends on how much is involved. Some parents have homes that have been downsized all along and are quick and easy to vacuum and dust. When surfaces of bathroom vanities, dressers, and kitchen counters aren't too cluttered, it may be a job you can also schedule to look after. Home care services offered through health departments or social services can be requested, and sometimes fees are subsidized based on income.

- <u>House Cleaning and Laundry Supplies:</u> All the laundry supplies were kept downstairs in the laundry room, with the iron and ironing board. A little drying rack was stored for use when items couldn't go in the dryer. One of our foreign workers needed more training as she put Mom's felt jacket in a hot water wash and it came out the size for a two-year-old! She felt bad. It happens. She learned.

Cleaning supplies were kept in a hall cupboard which had shallow shelves and enough room at the front for the brooms and dustpan. I purchased the clamps to install on the door for these, so they were kept off the floor and easier to get.

The shelves had cleaning supplies for typical surfaces of glass, chrome, tile, hardwood and polishing furniture. We had a disaster once when a foreign worker saw me polishing the furniture and used the same product on the floor. We then had to use an abrasive cleaner so we could safely walk on them again. Thank God, Mom and Dad wore rubber soled footwear, because I had a hard time staying upright in my stocking feet! Again, she felt bad. It happens. She learned.

Except for the vacuuming once a week, the live-in nurses did the light housekeeping without ever complaining, mostly when Mom and Dad were having their afternoon naps, and that only once a week. The rest of the time they could lie down on the "bunk" or the couch and rest or nap too.

- Good Waste Disposal Containers: I'm crazy about the odors in a house. After visiting seniors' facilities over the years with my pastor Dad, and then on my own, I can't tell if pet smells or odors from incontinence are worse. I also do everything I can to eliminate odors due to rotten food, or mildew. I would not have rented the house for Mom and Dad if I had smelled mildew when we first walked in.

This is how I had the waste containers figured out:

- Dry Waste: Bags, boxes, and dry items went in a large flip top lid bin. I measured the space between the wall and the fridge and purchased one that just fit there.
- Wet Kitchen Waste: Coffee grounds, tea bags, peels from fruits and vegetables all went into this container. It was attached to the cabinet door under the sink. It was lined with odor reducing bags and had a good fitting lid.

Linda McKendry

- <u>Sanitary Waste</u>: This was a small chrome, step-on, flip top container lined with a recycled grocery bag. It got filled with the used pull ups and the wipes or other non-flushables in the bathroom. This was emptied once a day into the main outdoor garbage bin by the back door.
- <u>Regular Waste</u>: Each room had small waste baskets within comfortable reach of beds or chairs for mostly facial tissues or light paper trash. Cookie wrappers. Dad's finished puzzle books... and the like.

These were collected on the house cleaning day and also put into the outside bin, along with everything from the rest of the house.

- <u>Yard Work</u>: In summer Joe mowed the lawn once a week and that was sufficient. One potted plant sat on the brick wall by the front door out of the way of the rail on the other side. It was easy to water and maintain. Mom and Dad both enjoyed it and commented when they entered and left the house.

In winter, between Joe and me, the snow on the driveway, sidewalks, and steps got shoveled. The front steps and the car got a sweep. Because we got an allowance from Veterans Affairs for this service, I made sure Joe was paid for what he did.

MEALS

- <u>Meals on Wheels</u>: Whether it's the formal organization, some other volunteer charity, or a benevolent group from your church or club who take meals to shut-ins and seniors, this is something that can be set up for your parents.

- Food Management: Shopping was done weekly with the weekly budget. This kept a nice supply of fresh fruits and vegetables. Discounts and sales were noted for the things we bought frequently like sugar-free puddings, ribs, oatmeal, peanut butter, etc.

We stocked up on a variety of small and medium fridge storage containers for preserving and serving prepared foods each day, or leftovers to be eaten the following day. I trained the foreign workers to prepare my parent's favorite foods in a nutritious and balanced way. They had it down to a science and we were all happy.

- Portion Control: Smaller portions all around. At the Lodge they got used to three meals and three snacks a day, so we made that part of the routine. If we were out for medical or hair appointments, even the grocery shopping, they were done around one of their "snack" times.
- Eating out: meant sharing one meal between the two of them. Since they had done this over the years and had similar favorites it was easy and economical. Mom would be the first to not eat everything, and Dad would be ready to finish whatever she didn't want.
- Nutrition: We instructed our foreign worker nurses to prepare meals with one protein, one carb, cooked vegetables with a hot meal, and raw vegetables with a sandwich or soup mostly for lunch. We rarely did salads with lettuce. It was easier to prepare and serve sliced cucumbers, celery, carrots, and zucchini. Little cups of salad dressing were enough for dipping or drizzling. Mom dipped. Dad drizzled!

Most desserts were a fruit cup with an arrowroot biscuit or a small bowl of frozen yogurt, sugar-free pudding, or oatmeal and raisin cookies. We never offered them anything made with white, refined flour or too much white sugar.

- <u>Medically Approved</u>: Dad was diabetic so he had some dietary restrictions. When he had a crisis and lost so much weight the dietician suggested cream in coffee and more toast with butter. As soon as his weight was increasing, we cut back on calories. When he had a DVT, certain foods were restricted, and his INR was tested more frequently. Mom ate far less and was pickier about her food. Dad liked flax seeds in his oatmeal. Mom didn't like the little "bugs" in hers and would obsess with picking them out. Dr. Cohen told me that often people with dementia obsess over their food. This was true for her.
- <u>Labels:</u> Labels were also important for communicating special instructions. I labeled many things so that there wouldn't be any confusion, and everyone could find things quickly and easily.

One example was the bottle of Lactaid Tabs. Mom was lactose intolerant but loved ice cream, whipping cream, and cream in her tea and coffee at the house. She wouldn't chew a Lactaid tablet, so I had drops too, in the house and the car.

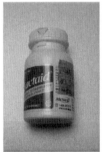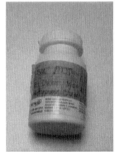

It says: "For MOM – 1 tab with ice cream, yogurt, or whipping cream (not milk)." Lactaid drops went into the milk jug. Another label!

MEDICAL

- Prescribed Drugs: We kept all medications and supplements on a single shelf in a special cupboard. The pharmacist put them in blister packs so it was easy to make sure they got what was prescribed each day: the proper dose, at the proper time.

When extra medication was being given for a temporary issue, especially strong pain relief, that had to be combined with stool softeners, I kept a journal on the counter. I would put in the recommended dose and note the time it was given. I also made a column for report of symptoms and side effects. Everyone on each shift was on top of the treatment. That gave me information I needed when reporting to doctors to stop or continue medications.

Due to depression and Mom's constant crying, there was a time when anti-depressants were prescribed. They weren't making any difference, so I asked the doctor how to wean her off them. Mom's sleeping pills were only given if she was restless and keeping Dad awake. Even then half a pill seemed to settle her down enough to go to sleep and still be able to use the washroom in the middle of the night safely.

- Activities: Dr. Yee sent Mom and Dad to an Occupational Therapy Clinic at the University. Dad could do his on the bed right after breakfast. He wouldn't do them before he got out of bed because eating "for strength to do them" was the first thing on his mind each day. His were for his hip joint function and strength.

Linda McKendry

Mom's required that we get permission from the landlord to install a small pulley over a door in the hallways. She then had a rope with knots at the right place so when she pulled down with one arm the other arm would rise. She also had an elastic strap that attached to a doorknob to be pulled forwards and backwards. This was to strengthen the ligaments and muscles in her shoulders.

- First Aid Items and Medications Safe: First Aid items, such as the blood pressure monitor, thermometer, and small wound care were kept with the ostomy supplies.

Prescription drugs and supplements, like Vitamin C, were kept in little baskets on top of the fridge. One for Mom and one for Dad. Each one had the blister packs from the pharmacist and any additional supplements they might be taking. Dad's also had his blood sugar monitor, supplies, and logbook which he used each morning before eating.

We kept logs consistent with their daily routines to make realistic comparisons. As I mentioned, when either of them was taking temporary medications for treatment of a condition I kept a journal/log book on the counter so each shift knew what was happening and when the last dose had been given. Now I would do this on an electronic device. You never need to have a pen handy!

MOOD

- State of Mind: Dr. Cohen would always ask them, and then me, "How's your mood?" We refer to people as being "moody" when they are up and down emotionally. Mom and Dad were pretty even-tempered, and even symptoms of dementia were predictable based on the circumstances.

- Emotional Health: We never knew with Dad if he was content or depressed. He would carry around his Word Search Puzzle books and be ready to do another one anywhere and anytime. He never acknowledged Mom's condition and many times treated her like he expected her to do what she had always done.

We were constantly on his case trying to explain Mom's condition and he would nod and just go back to his puzzles, watching TV, or having his snack. He was the first to suggest each day that we should go out for some fresh air. This meant get out of the house, a ride in the car, pick up a newspaper, get drive-through coffee, and take it to a park or lake.

- Well-being: I feel that because we kept routines in place and everything on the calendar, Dad was able to check on what he could look forward to each day, or on the weekend.

Mom was just content to be by his side and get as close as she could without him chiding her and teasing her, "Did you want to sit on my lap?" Her wellbeing was almost entirely based on if he was in her view and doing okay. Even when she suffered a couple of falls, broken ribs in one case, and undiagnosed in the other, she was still concerned about where her "Johnny" was.

- Mean Streaks: Dementia and their own frustrations and confusion can cause mean streaks. To us it felt like Dad was being mean to Mom all the time because of his expectations and teasing. We were constantly explaining to him why she couldn't or wouldn't be able to accommodate him. Dad would send her to the kitchen to get him a cup of coffee. We'd find her there wandering around and not knowing what to do. Dad would holler, "What's taking you so long, Lydia? Have you gone to Calcutta?" This would make her laugh but didn't help her make the coffee. From time to time, she would come and find the caregiver on duty and say, "Johnny wants a cup of coffee." And then go back to her chair beside him. When she did this, we weren't sure if Dad had given her that instruction or she had figured it out on her own. I'm still not sure, but it was better.

Mom's mean streaks were only directed at the nurses or medical personnel trying to get her to do something to get a diagnosis. One time we could not get her to give a urine sample. She declared that was plain stupid. Other times I would don a lead apron in order to stand close to Mom in the X-ray room and coax her to do what they needed. This was especially important when we suspected she had fractured ribs from a fall.

Her pedicurist and hairdresser were both threatened by her if she didn't like something they were doing. Because of their extreme patience and figuring out ways to make Mom happy, I always budgeted for generous tips. I often wondered what would have happened to her if she had been all alone in a facility with so many strangers around her trying to help her. There's no doubt in my mind she would have had to be medicated or restrained. The thought of that makes me eternally grateful she had us there to comfort her and prevent any meltdowns.

Dementia? Or normal frustration? All of us react to situations negatively when we are triggered. In traffic with aggressive drivers. In stores where clerks are rude. With companies when we make a purchase that needs to be fixed or returned. We are all likely to have our moments and we can't expect our parents or seniors to be any different.

I was always careful to determine if any mean streak was due to dementia or normal frustration before judging or taking permanent action, as in the case of Mom's treatment of the nurses, which I believe was the dementia. Dad's was more of frustration, but the dementia maybe had an effect on his level of denial of Mom's condition.

MONEY

- Cash on Hand. I kept cash on hand with the monthly grocery budget when I had others helping to pick up the groceries. Because our nurses didn't drive, I would have a friend pick them all up and take them to the grocery store. She would drop off the nurse at the supermarket, and then take Mom and Dad for coffee. They would all come back with groceries, receipts, and change. Dad was happy to pay for coffee and snacks out of his allowance.
- Paying Expenses. I set aside one Friday morning a month to pay the bills. They all got tucked in one place near my desk. Some had auto debit arranged but most were paid by check. The household expenses had to be kept separate from the expenses paid for by the Self Managed Care Funding. I could use the funds to pay someone to come and take Mom and Dad out or shopping, so that was tracked for their audits.
- Managing the Budget. I managed the budget by identifying our fixed costs that were the same each month. The rent and utilities were always the same. Electricity and gas varied

throughout the year, but in the first year I noted the maximum and budgeted for that.

I always calculated the tithe first and divided that by the number of weekends so Dad could have an offering to take to church. This was important to him and the charitable tax receipt at the year's end reduced his taxes which was good all around. I budgeted for one meal a month at a restaurant so we could still go out. This covered mine and Joes' too. If we didn't get out during the week I would cover the cost of weekend brunch after church for which ever sibling and spouse was on duty.

Dad's allowance came from dividing up the amount of interest from what we took every six months to subsidize income. Each Friday I would drive through the bank and hand him the cash which he happily put into his wallet and asked who would be driving him to the garage sales. Having some cash in his wallet was important to him and we felt that it increased his self-esteem and independence in that area.

MOBILITY

- Exercise: Move to move! You must keep moving so bones, muscles, and ligaments don't seize up. Mobility is always part of medical assessment and especially for home care. Mobility also requires more attention to safety and having good strong support to hold on to and guide over curbs and downstairs.

There is a right way to support someone with your arm tucked into theirs inside their elbow. If you are just holding their hand, the strength may not be there if a fall happens.

Done With Dementia

There is risk to injuring a limb with no stability for the entire body or balance in a moment's notice.

There are aids to daily living such as proper canes, walkers, and transport or wheelchairs. A visit with a good therapist will show your parents how to walk and get in and out of chairs safely. Dad once dived for his chair instead of backing up to it until he could feel his legs against the seat. He ended up fracturing some of his ribs! Even then we had to constantly remind him to back into a chair, always looking for the armchair in a waiting room or restaurant.

- Appropriate Physical Activity: Dad had a little exercise bike that we traded up for an elliptical. He would also go for walks around the house in circles through the kitchen, dining room, living room and hallway.

We would give shoppers a shock when we turned up at the mall with Mom sitting in the transport chair and Dad pushing her, only to have them trade places and she would push him. This was a win-win for all of us especially when there were no places to stop and sit down to rest.

- Handicap Parking: Regulations for this differ from place to place. For us, a doctor fills out a form used to apply for the rear-view mirror tag at vehicle registration offices. The tag is for the passenger, not the vehicle. Whoever your parent is traveling with can use it. We had one for each of our parents and two vehicles, so we just kept one of their tags in each car. There are fines if the tag is checked against the ID for the passengers. We decided not to worry about that since most of the time we had both parents in the car together.

- Capsule of Life: This is available at some pharmacies, fire stations, or EMS departments. A doctor fills out the form and endorses the conditions explained. It details the level of life support to be given based on the cause of the emergency and condition of the parent. DNR is the code for "Do Not Resuscitate." A list of the residents' prescriptions is included for diagnosis of some conditions. These documents roll up and fit into a metal cigar-sized tube. It is kept in the freezer door with a bright fluorescent pink fridge magnet logo.

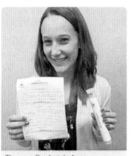
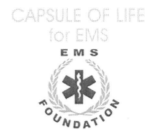

CAPSULE OF LIFE
for EMS

Therese Frederick, former administrative co-ordinator for the EMS Foundation, holds up a sheet of paper to be completed with a person's medical information. It is then rolled up, placed in a Capsule of Life and stored in the person's refrigerator where emergency personnel can easily find it in the event of an emergency.

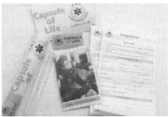

- Call Buttons: These are attached to a senior's body either as a wrist band or a pendant to wear around the neck. If someone has a fall, it will alert an emergency line that will either talk to the injured or confused wearer, and/or immediately send for EMS ambulance. Most facilities we visited had emergency pull cords logically placed by beds, easy chairs, and in bathrooms. These are wired to a main central desk, but there are call buttons made for individuals in their own homes too.

Dementia Disclaimer: Unfortunately, someone with dementia doesn't benefit from wearing a call button. Firstly, they won't remember to keep it on, even though many are designed to be worn 24/7 including in the bath or shower. Secondly, if they take it off or throw it onto a bed or table, it can activate as if the person has fallen and alert the EMS. In my mother's case, she had a nice long chat with a man she never saw, whose company she was delighted with. He kept her company until Dad returned home. It was just one more thing that alerted us to the level of dementia.

- Area Rugs: Area rugs are considered a tripping hazard and I have mixed feelings about them. I do believe your parents should have comfortable indoor shoes, or closed back, rubber sole slippers to wear in the house. I put down rubber backed mud mats from the threshold of the front door and down the hall almost to where it turned. This mat had a rubber flange all around the sides and would never curl. It kept mud, snow, and salt off the hardwood floors and gave a lot of space for them to walk well inside the house to give us room to close the door.

I also kept the area rug in the living room after watching them walk on and off the edge of it. My reasoning was partly aesthetics, but also to minimize the noise and coldness of the floors. The mats I purchased for their bedsides were also very flat, rubber backed and didn't curl. These were removed when Mom began to spit and throw up due to severe indigestion. Accidents from incontinence were easier to clean up on the floor than on a bedside rug. Dad was having leaks from his bag or missing the pee pot he kept by the bed at night. It became more of a sanitary issue than a safety one, but I was still aware of the hazard of scatter mats. In the bathroom we had a tub mat for both inside and outside the tub which was only put down during bath time.

- Furniture Walking: Watch to see if your parents are doing what is called "furniture walking" where they reach for one piece of furniture after another in order to navigate and keep their balance. This is dangerous, as some items if not stable and secure can tip or move and cause a fall and injury.

Chairs especially need to have rubber castors to prevent them moving as your parent is getting up or sitting down in a chair. Arms are very important to provide guidance and support. Casters with teeth are available to dig into carpet and area rugs to keep furniture from sliding.

MENTORING

- Guiding. You will always be mentoring your parents and this is where the "parenting your parents" comes in. They need guidance throughout the day and sometimes into the night too. You are there to do that.
- Encouraging. They still need encouragement. When they do something well, don't feel shy to clap, or say thanks, and act excited about their accomplishments.
- Challenging. After Dad's medical crisis when he had to learn to walk all over again, we watched therapists at the rehab center challenge him when he wanted to quit or stop too soon. We learned to push him a little at home to keep up the good work. I couldn't let myself get lazy either when I wasn't in the mood to remind Dad of therapy exercises and set them up for him.

We were challenged with Mom to keep her from sitting and crying for hours at a time. We could stop the tears with distractions like her favorite movie or Gospel music DVDs. Sometimes asking her to play the keyboard was enough to get her out of her funk.

- <u>Inspiring</u>. Mom would often read words on a sign or wall plaque over and over again. I used that to my advantage and taped some positive confessions on the walls in the bathroom, opposite the toilet, and where she would see them in the living room. The letters needed to be big enough to read across the room! My purpose was to have her hear what she was reading and hopefully be influenced by the positive message at some level.

MOTHERING

- <u>Grooming</u>: Dad did his own grooming. He shaved with an electric shaver, brushed his teeth, and soaked his dentures at night. He had a shower each time the ileostomy bag had to be changed, which averaged once a week. He used deodorant and combed his hair all day with a comb stuck in his shirt pocket.

Mom, on the other hand, had to be guided for all her grooming. She could hold her hairbrush in one hand, while using the other hand for support under her elbow to fix her hair. We had to assist her to brush her teeth by handing her the toothbrush with paste on it. We'd hand her a washcloth with the soap and then help with rinsing and drying. She had perms regularly at first, but after her last fall she was too weak and uncooperative, so we had her hair cut in a short, straight style easy for us to manage.

- <u>Dressing</u>: Dad dressed himself and always wore a button-down shirt and dress pants. We had to purchase extra-large pants and modify the length so they could be worn with suspenders to accommodate the bulge of the ileostomy bag as it filled. He refused to wear the stretch track pants he came home from the hospital in and changed to slacks as soon as possible. He always looked the part of a gentleman and a minister!

He didn't need any help to pick the right coat or his hat. He did need reminding from time to time to not leave his hat behind in restaurants, or in church. Mom needed help to dress all the time. Not because she was feeble or weak, but because she didn't remember to dress and couldn't make appropriate decisions for the climate or activity.

- Directions: We erred on the side of over explaining and directing to guide them along throughout the day and night. This was like parenting a small child all day. We got used to saying the same thing over and over again. The difference is that we didn't expect them to learn it on their own or remember.

Like many experts in elder care will tell you, when they have dementia, you don't ask them if they want their lunch. You say, "Come, Mom, it's time for lunch." And you guide them to the table. There's no point in asking them to make a choice or a decision, and sometimes they don't know where to go exactly, so you gently and firmly take their arm and lead them.

- Choices: As already stated, you can see that we had to make a lot of choices for them. Therefore what you learn when you take the survey will help you give them what they are used to or prefer. This doesn't mean that you never give them a choice either. If we had more than one flavor of fruit cup, or cookie, we would give them a choice. Again, Dad was more engaged in this and would sometimes even say, "Can I have one of each?"

Mom, when given a choice of watching a movie or a Gospel concert on a video, would often say, "I don't care. I like them all." But even this answer told us she was in a reasonable state of reality.

MEMORY

- Reminders: Daily reminders, like telling them what day of the week it was, or what routine event they had just enjoyed was something done ongoing. Many times, a sentence would begin with, "Remember? Today we are going to the clinic." We knew that Dad would take this into account and be planning, looking forward to an outing with coffee or lunch. He also wanted to know if he would still get his afternoon nap.

Whenever Mom made a move to get up and go somewhere, we would just follow her and gauge if she needed help or not since she still did a few things on her own.

- Stories from Past: As is often the case, your parents will remember vivid details from their past or their childhood, yet not remember a few minutes back. Dad told stories and had memories we could confirm by having heard many tales of his past from his siblings and from our own experience growing up with them.

Mom, on the other hand, never spoke of their time in India, didn't kibitz in the Indian language which we all spoke as a family, and never spoke of their time in Canada in the pastorate. She repeatedly told stories of being a girl on the farm. She spoke of playing duets with her father on a single guitar. She talked about the blocks of ice they would bring up from the frozen creek in the winter with horses to line a straw-bale pit that they used to keep food cold all summer. She loved to talk about her mother, who would approach strangers on the farm with a rifle in her hand, and of all the DIY veterinarian treatments she did for their farm animals and those of their neighbors. I would listen with delight at these stories and could write a whole book on them. These confirmed to me a level of reality from her past that she still remembered.

This, however, made her decide to go and visit her parents one day. Josie, the nurse, called to let me know Mom was outside, in winter, with just her nightgown and slippers, refusing to come in because she had to go to her parents. Josie had her cornered on the neighbor's deck and I called my daughter to go over there as soon as possible until I could get there. After that we had a lock put high on the entrance doors, front and back to prevent her from just wandering outside. That didn't stop her from continuing to want to see them. Any reminder that they had passed away didn't seem to register or change her mind.

- Familiar Things: Keep as many familiar things around them as possible. We purposely kept artwork, framed family photos, and ornaments in the rooms they sat in for hours each day. We also had all the photo albums my mother had so carefully made with titles, dates, and each photo labelled.

At first, we would give one to Mom to look at and she would sit for hours, turning the pages and making comments. We would pay attention to whether she remembered the people or not. She'd always remember "my Johnny" and her sister, her parents, and some of us kids or places they had visited. But many times, she'd just make general comments about the people or things in the pictures as if they belonged to someone else.

The day came when she began to take out the pictures and then just put them back in any album, in any place. She would also lose interest and not look at them for any length of time. We stopped giving them to her at that time, unless we were sitting next to her and going through, pointing out individuals and telling her about them. She'd nod and enjoy the process, but none of these stimulated her memory.

MAIN THINGS

- <u>The Mandate</u>: Remember your big promise! Whatever you decide is the main reason to keep your parents together is probably written in stone. We didn't go to all the trouble to make and keep a home for them 24/7 just to let it all go when we got tired or frustrated.

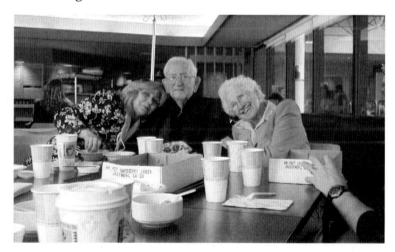

- <u>Moments of Truth</u>: There will be moments of truth, both good and bad. Many will tell you that that person you have always known as your mother, or your father, is still there. Other times you will be dismayed or discouraged as you see them suffering even more from aging or dementia changing the person you have always known.

- <u>May not come to stay</u>: There are some things that may not come to stay. You must be prepared for all the changes. Each time we experienced an accident that caused temporary injury and were dealing with the symptoms during the healing process, it often felt like this was a lifetime sentence… for them and for us. Bodies are resilient, especially when cared for and loved unconditionally. Some form of physical health usually returned.

- <u>Mercy and Patience</u>: both go a long way in a day. I am often reminded of the Bible verse that says, "Blessed are the merciful, for they shall obtain mercy." Knowing the amount of mercy I need causes me to extend more mercy towards others. Most people, I included, don't do aggravating things on purpose!

MAGIC OF LOVE

- <u>Firm, but Gentle Touch</u>: This is so important especially when physically helping and guiding your parent. There is a difference between grabbing someone's arm in an abusive way and gently, but firmly, gripping their arm to let them know you've got a safe hold on them. This is also important when helping someone bath, dry off, or clean their bottom. Too light a touch may feel ticklish or cause the skin to itch. Too firm may hurt skin that is delicate and thin. Pay attention to body language that reveals discomfort and make adjustments.

- <u>Endearing Words</u>: Experts in dementia care will tell you that sometimes a person can't understand what you are saying, but they respond to the tone of voice and your expression. Isn't this true for all of us? I'm guilty of just blurting out what I feel needs to be said with frequent lack of paying attention to the tone of my voice. Occasionally I would see the startled expression on my parents' faces, especially if we needed to do something urgently. I would repeat myself with a softer tone, or even say I was sorry for saying it that way. They immediately responded positively to that as well! You must learn to have a soft tone while still being loud enough for them to hear you clearly. My husband is suffering with some hearing loss after an aneurysm on his brain and I find myself shouting to make myself heard, and even I don't like the tone of my voice.

When my mother was feeling threatened by a nurse trying to put in a catheter, or a hygienist trying to clean her teeth, I would get close to her, get her attention if I could, and say, "I love you!" with huge emphasis on the word "love." She couldn't resist smiling and saying, "I love you too." Then I could explain what the person helping her was trying to do and why. She seemed to calm down and grab my hand and squeeze it for reassurance. Each time the staff expressed gratitude that I was there to make their job easier.

- <u>Loving Look into Their Eyes</u>: In my opinion, this is even more important than the tone of voice. Put the two together and you have a winning, and winsome, combination. My parents were always looking into my eyes for the truth of what I was saying.

The one time I know I had a mean look in my eyes, because of how I was feeling, my mother reacted immediately by looking away and then looking down. I realized what I had done and I immediately told her I loved her and gave her a hug. When she looked up at me, I could tell she wasn't quite sure. But she came back to looking at me with that little sparkle and smile of recognition in her eyes.

She often referred to me as "my mother" when people came to the house, or we were out and about. This amused me because it was obvious why she would think that.

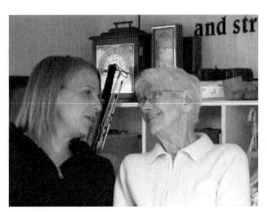

In this picture I took of my daughter Kim and my mother enjoying some time in the sun porch, you can see what a good time they are having. Kim often said, "I know grandma doesn't remember my name. But I think she knows me on some level."

IF YOU FIND LACK IN FLOW CONSIDER MY THREE RULES...

RULE #1: Have a plan.

RULE #2: Be flexible.

RULE #3: Perform other duties as required.

If a plan isn't working, don't let it become the "tail wagging the dog." Modify the routine, schedule, space or storage, or make a new plan. Go back to rule #1.

Advise those helping and explain the changes. Care and comfort of parents is priority. If something isn't working invite those helping to make suggestions. Sometimes they can have flexibility and modify what they do when they are on duty and it isn't going to affect much in the big picture. If they prefer to poach eggs rather than fry them, for example, it's no big deal.

On other occasions, I had to explain again to everyone why something was particularly important to be done a certain way for a certain reason or it would throw everything and everyone else off. I made it clear that bringing in certain foods would cause Mom to have constipation and we were avoiding that at all costs. Dad's blood sugar was a concern as well. So, we all worked to pay attention to the important stuff and be flexible about the not-so-important stuff. It was a process.

ENJOY YOUR PARENTS AS PART OF YOUR LIFE

DEATH: DONE-WITH-DEMENTIA

Mom Leaves Dad

The hardest chapter to write in this book is about the circumstances leading up to Mom's death. She had been losing weight consistently, about one pound a month for eighteen months. She was checked by the different doctors and there didn't appear to be anything causing it except that she ate like a bird. She'd perk right up when her favorite things were offered and appear to have a good appetite but then she'd leave a lot of food and we were constantly coaxing her to eat.

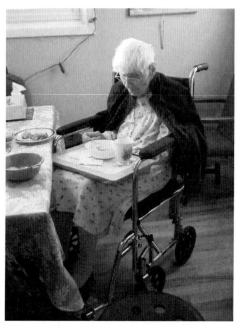

One of our foreign nurses who had worked for a time in a large facility told us of one woman who was kept alive on a popular meal replacement drink for two years. I checked into the label on the drink and decided there weren't enough natural or nutritious ingredients, and in fact, the list contained ingredients being warned about and suspect of causing disease. (You can look them up for yourself and judge.) Mom was still mobile and energetic for her age. She never complained about walks or planned activities. Our main challenge with her ongoing was the length of time she would just sit and cry. Most of our distractions worked but she never complained about being tired either, or even sad about anything. I personally wondered if Dad's nose in his puzzle books all the time was affecting her and she felt rejection, but that couldn't be proved.

One night while I was on duty, I heard a crash and flipped on the light as I dashed into their bedroom. Mom was collapsed on the floor at the foot of the bed on Dad's side. She had somehow either fainted or run into something that knocked her out. She was between the bed and Dad's dresser. I ran to grab the phone and called 911. I asked Dad to throw me her pillow so I could put it under her head. She wasn't bleeding or cut. I called out to her, "Mom, are you okay? Mom! Mom! Lydia… Lydia!"

I don't remember when she came to. The ambulance was there in five minutes and they immediately picked her up and put her on the bed, began to do her vitals and hook her up to the EKG. I do remember her opening her eyes, blinking with a confused look and a little scowl on her face. I reassured her about what was happening. I was waiting for her to make some mean remark about them hurting her or accusing them of being naughty if they were touching a private part of her body. But they took over in their professional manner and I just backed off.

I knew this would be a trip to the hospital and I had to figure out what to do for Dad's care. I called the landlord, who was then living in the apartment downstairs after Joe moved out. I asked if he would come up until my daughter could get there. He was up in a flash and I rode in the front of the ambulance to the hospital. The ambulance attendants seemed to understand that because of her dementia she would be easier to deal with if accompanied by me. I praised God for that especially after Dad had been re-routed to a different hospital when the ambulance had taken him last. Even if I had to follow the ambulance in my car, I wasn't going to let it out of my sight.

At the hospital, they hooked her up to all the emergency monitoring equipment and that included a catheter. She was immediately upset and told them how bad they were to be touching her there. I held her hands up to her chest and leaned over smiling into her face and telling her how much I loved her. She nodded at me and smiled back, which was just enough distraction for them to complete the task. Upon examination they found extreme pain in her side and believed she might have fractured ribs or bruised organs. I couldn't tell them what had caused the fall or if she had just fainted. I often wondered if she was heading the wrong way to the washroom, heading towards the night light plugged into the wall on Dad's side of the bed and ran right into it. She usually walked with a slight stoop so she would have hit the top of her head, but that wasn't where her pain was. It was in her right side.

The next challenge in the hospital was getting her down for an x-ray. In this case too, I had to don a lead vest in order to help her get into the position they needed. Her confusion, lack of cooperation, and resisting not moving for even a second resulted in getting her back to bed as soon as possible. I know they would have had to sedate her if I hadn't been there. The x-rays were clear enough to reveal no broken bones and no major internal issues.

She was given extra strength Tylenol, which was also a challenge to get her to take, and an IV to keep her hydrated. I slept in the lounge chair next to her and we both slept relatively peacefully considering the other cases being treated on each side of the curtains. In the morning after a tray of porridge and toast, coffee and orange juice, they determined she should just go home, rest, and take the prescribed pain killers as required. I called my husband to come and get us and asked him to stop by the house and pick up her street clothes, shoes, and a winter coat.

We chatted in the entrance to the hospital as we waited, and she was unusually bright and talkative. She was tickled to see Jim.

Hugged him and thanked him profusely for driving her home.

Erin our student nurse was on duty and I know she can verify what happened next. Mom's younger sister who lives in Texas called. We listened while they had the most amazing conversation with Mom just explaining everything as if she had never lost her memory. She was in a bright mood, laughing and like her old self. I was stunned! She falls, we take her to the hospital, she has one overnight stay, gets majorly hydrated, takes some Tylenol Three and she's brighter than she's ever been. From that moment on I did everything I could to get her to drink more.

Her pain increased to where none of the pain medication was helping. Getting her to move at all for dressing or coming to the table was excruciating for her. I got out the transport chair to use in the house to help her get from room to room. I also brought a portable potty with arms and pushed it into the side of the closet by her bed, so she didn't have to go far for the washroom. Within days we just had confusion and chaos. Her doctor was on holidays and I couldn't get Dr. Cohen's office because it was Christmas break at the University. I couldn't convince her it was okay to just pee in her pull ups in the bed or the chair. Helping her up to stand or walk was a huge cry of pain.

I reasoned after breakfast one day that I should try and help Mom get from the transport chair into her easy chair since she would be there most of the day and we could bring her food in there on a tray if necessary. As I lifted her up to swivel her body into the easy chair, she bit me on my chest just above my right breast. The shock of it made me drop her back into the chair like a sack of potatoes. I ran down the hall into the bedroom. I called my sister in a flood of tears, and told her what had happened. I asked her to come and help me. She had offered so many times and now I felt exhausted from all day and all-night vigil over Mom.

To prevent another fall, I had ordered an alarm mat that goes on a patient's bed and if they get up it sets off an alarm. The landlord gave permission for me to run the wire from the mat through the closet wall into the caregiver's room so it would go off there and not in Mom and Dad's room. It never got used. By the time Susie came, we had Mom moved into the hospital bed in the other room so we could raise and lower it to make helping her easier on both of us.

While Susie gave me a whole night of complete rest in my own bed at home, I spent some time calling around to see if I could get Mom hydrated again. It seemed to me that she just needed this while she recovered from internal bruises since that's all that seemed to be diagnosed.

My niece had been given a portable IV, so she didn't have to stay in the hospital for treatment. I reasoned we could do the same for Mom. Having a catheter would also make attempts at helping her go to the bathroom not so painful for her. I was told to just take her to the emergency, explain the situation, and see what they could do. I called a cab for wheelchair access and called Susie with my plan to take Mom to the hospital.

Susie did her best to dress Mom and help her use the portable potty, again with a lot of pain. We helped her into the transport chair instead of back into bed. Even as I helped her down the front steps and into the cab, Adan's mom was pulling into the driveway to drop him off. Mom whimpered all the way to the hospital and then groaned constantly in the half empty waiting room. The triage nurse didn't see much need to move Mom too quickly because there were no beds available in any of the suitable wards. Finally, Mom was taken into emergency and set up there. This part of the emergency department had walls instead of curtains dividing the beds. As we went through the same antics of inserting a catheter and IV's in Mom's arm, she finally settled into resting and sleeping. A couple of times she would reach over pat my arm, and say, "My darling. I'm so glad you are here!" They brought in a portable ultrasound machine to see if they could determine what was causing so much pain in her side. I stayed the night with Mom, and it was the best rest I'd had in a long time. I was right about the catheter and hydrating combined. The nurses brought me a lounge bed chair, warmed flannel sheets, and a pillow. I would open an eye from time to time as the nurses came in to check on us, and it was comforting to look over at Mom sleeping peacefully.

In the morning Susie came to take my place and give me a break. Erin was on duty at the house with Dad so my husband came to take me home. Before I left, Susie and I had a discussion with a nurse and after that her IV was turned off and she was changed to palliative care. I left the hospital with a very heavy heart. I had brought Mom in to help her get better and now she was going to die. It was just a matter of time with palliative care treatment. I released her to Susie because I was too tired to argue or plead my case anymore. But because I was the EPOA it was up to me to say if the IV was turned off or not. Reluctantly I agreed... against everything in my heart. To this day I question my lack of strength to stand up and resist the reasons being given to me even though they were logical. I called the family to let them know Mom was in the hospital and in palliative care, which means a vigil has started as a loved one is considered terminal.

The Angel of Death: At one point we were all gathered in the lobby of the emergency except Dad who was with Erin. I suddenly had this urge to call her to bring Dad over to see Mom. While we were waiting in the lobby, I noticed a lady, very pale, wearing black who had jet black hair sitting in the corner and apparently not waiting for anyone. She was watching our family encounters and each of us thought one of us knew her. Just after I called the nurse to bring Dad over, she came up to me and said, "It won't be long now for your loved one." And she walked out of the front door of the hospital. We all looked at each other and asked, "Who was that? Did you know her?" I took comfort in her words and it confirmed my sudden decision to have Dad come as soon as possible.

The Final Family Meeting with Mom.

When Dad arrived, I asked the emergency nurses if we could all come in for a few minutes, to just surround Mom's bed... that we would be very quiet coming in and not make any disturbance. They had asked us about moving her to a Hospice, but we decided we didn't want to do palliative care at home when we found out what was involved. At this sudden request, they first reminded me they were trying to find a bed in a ward, and then we could all visit her there. But for some reason they changed their mind when

I told them we had some family from out of town who were just traveling through and had to leave soon. And Dad was on his way.

I also believe that because it was one of the rooms with walls, they were more cooperative in letting us all come in. I explained to the family that I would lead the way. We were to walk quietly and quickly, not stay more than five minutes and then leave the same way. As soon as Dad arrived, we made our way into Mom's bedside. The nurses had moved Mom's bed clear to the back of the space and smoothed it out. I hadn't seen Mom since I had left her with Susie earlier that day and I was shocked at her appearance. She was already gaunt; her skin was very pale and tight to the bones. She had her mouth open and her eyes closed but was breathing slowly and evenly. As everyone gathered around, I went up to her, leaned over and said, "Mom. We are all here to have a prayer with you. Dad is here too." She didn't nod or respond in any way. I asked Erin to put Dad's transport chair next to her on one side and then we lined ourselves up in a circle around the room.

I can't remember some of the details, except I wish we had recorded Susie's prayer. It was one that thanked God for the mother He had given us, for her love and legacy, and she committed Mom into His hands. When she faltered a bit, Jim said he squeezed her hand and she was able to continue with a strong voice. We all knew it might be the last time we saw her alive, but it was up to God. I asked everyone to leave so Dad could have a few minutes alone with Mom.

I peeked in to see him lay his hand on Mom's arm and repeat the Aaronic blessing over her. "The Lord bless you and keep you. The Lord make His face to shine upon you. The Lord lift His countenance upon you and give you peace. Amen." I don't know if he kissed her or if he knew how close to death she was. He didn't express any emotion. We left and Susie was arranging for her daughter to come and sit with Mom so she could have a break.

Jim and I left to pick up pizza and salads so we could all have lunch together back at the house. When I walked into the house, my brother met me at the door. "Susie called. Mom's gone." Dad was sitting in his chair and I knelt at his side and wept. He laid his hands on my head but didn't say anything. When I looked up, he was just nodding. Susie had retreated to the caregiver's bedroom. She didn't want to come out and have the family meeting we needed to decide what to do next. I told her that if she didn't come out, we would all come in there!

We weren't prepared for Mom to pass away so soon. Susie had revealed that at Mom's last breath she had opened her eyes and they were the bluest blue Susie had ever seen, and then she took her last breath. Susie said she died quietly and peacefully, so that was a comfort to all of us. We knew she was with her Lord and Savior. It was December 21st, 2012, the winter solstice: the day all the ancient calendars ended. Her calendar ended that day too. We lightened our grief by making note that Mom would spend Christmas in heaven with Jesus himself! We then began to make plans for her funeral or memorial service. We made a few phone calls and a list of what we had to arrange.

We turned to Dad a few times to get his input. He just nodded in agreement at what we were planning. He agreed with our plans for the location and the order of service. My brother noted that we were supposed to take the garments for Mom to be buried to the funeral home.

My daughter Kim had made a flannel nightgown for Mom for Christmas that had pockets in it for the tissues Mom always carried around. It was in a gift bag under their Christmas tree for one of us to pick up.

Gary and Janice had bought her a cozy fleece blanket to cover up with because she often complained of having cold legs. We decided to dress her in her new nightgown with a fresh tissue in one pocket, her little New Testament Bible in the other pocket, her reading glasses, her teeth, her hearing aids, her burgundy slippers, fresh pull ups, and pretty socks. Then the fleece throw would cover her too. Even though we never had an open casket, we were comforted by knowing how she would be laid to rest. We were all in agreement and that's what mattered.

Ironically, the amount of money I had saved for her to have dental surgery, which we were told was inevitable, was what we needed for the down payment on her casket and funeral. Susie came with me to pick it out. Mom and Dad always joked about being buried in a pine box so with Dad's approval, we picked a beautifully finished pine casket. It was only for the graveside service, which we arranged for the first Saturday in January. I also arranged for my daughter's sister-in-law, who does photography, to hover over the services and take candid pictures. My main reason was so I could send them to Mom's sister in Texas, knowing she would not be able to make it for the celebrations of Mom's life. A video would have captured the beautiful words of Scripture, prayers, our singing, and last words as we said a final goodbye.

We laid Mom to rest under the trees in the most beautiful cemetery overlooking the Rockies to the west, and now our parents were no longer together.

Linda McKendry

Dad Without Mom

Only 69 Days Apart

So now I deviate from the topic of keeping your parents together, but we still had a parent we wanted to see comfortable at home. We kept a watchful eye on Dad with nearly constant company. None of us ever saw any outward evidence of grief and thought maybe Dad had made peace with their inevitable home going. However, Susie remarked that when she went in to change Dad's bag at night, Dad's head was way over towards Mom's side of the bed. When Dad was in hospital, we girls had slept in the bed with Mom on Dad's side so we could be there for her especially when she constantly asked "Where's my Johnny?". No one was sleeping with Dad.

At Mom's memorial service, which was held just down the road from the cemetery, we saw Dad "holding court" as everyone came to express their condolences. He was smiling, thanking them and remembering many as parishioners, pastoral colleagues, friends, family, and neighbors. We used this occasion for some family photo ops. Dad's siblings. Our cousins. We used the transport chair and Erin was there to assist him and empty his bag as required. He also had his cane so he could walk around if he wanted to. The trouble was he began to use it to "nudge" people out of the way who were in front of him as he was being transported. I, my daughter, and my sister-in-law each chided him and asked him to not do that.

All during the service, the reception, and afterwards, no one saw any expression of sadness or emotion of grief. I had learned that he held in a lot for himself, even though he gave so much, including illustrations in sermons that he shared with emotion that would bring his congregation to tears. Everyone loved him. He joked and laughed a lot, teased, and always had stickers in his coat pocket for kids who ran up to him or came to sit on his lap in church. He could be serious at the religious ceremonies and always had appropriate behavior. But I also knew that he couldn't open up to some things that were personal or extra sensitive. We didn't pressure him.

Where to Live Now

Gary and Janice agreed to take Dad to their farm as he was stable and only in need of food, shelter, ostomy supplies, and his puzzle books. We had put Dad on the waiting list at the Colonel Belcher Veterans Assisted Living Facility. They had told us the wait might be three months. Gary and Janice would take Dad for a short time before they left for a holiday, and then we would decide which of us he could stay with. Susie had offered their home. I knew I could also have him stay with us for a short time, even though I was now facing Jim's heart surgery for an aneurism. God would make a way! But God had other plans. Dad's name came up after three weeks instead of three months. We had to decide.

After Mom passed away, it was instantly obvious that we couldn't continue to keep Dad in the house we had rented. Looking back, we should have used their available finances to keep Dad there a bit longer. And we didn't know what would transpire for him to move so soon after Mom's death. Because he was a veteran, he qualified to be a resident in the Colonel Belcher Retirement complex. I called and applied after we took Dad for a tour. Like the meetings we had in their original home when pressured to decide about moving, he nodded in agreement and understanding, but didn't smile.

Linda McKendry

I assumed they would realize he was more independent and mobile than some of the residents and we didn't think they would place him in a lockdown ward where he wouldn't be able to go out to the coffee bar, buy a newspaper, or navigate the complex on his own. The scariest thing for me was that I had to sign off on making any medical decisions because there was a doctor assigned to the complex. They did reassure me that I would be consulted about the choices and have a say in what was decided for him. They also demanded that he get a flu shot, which we didn't do as a matter of principle, seeing how many people still got severe cases of flu even when they had the shot. However, living alone in our environment compared to a more public place meant Dad would be exposed to more germs and viruses. I had to give in on that one too.

Susie had stayed back even after Dad was in the Colonel, partly to stay with him during the day and partly to help me clean out the house since we had given our required notice to the landlord. She noticed things at the facility that bothered her. I'm not detailing some of what we witnessed for sake of liability, but I'd put it down to not enough staff on hand, in the right place at the right time.

One thing I noticed when I went early one morning was that a pair of Dad's dress pants was sitting on a chair with the inseam exposed and all covered with a white cream. Dad was already down having breakfast, so I went to find him. When I inquired with one of the staff why his pants had cream in the seat, I was told that they automatically do that for all the residents because most of them sit all day. Apparently, it was to prevent pressure sores. We explained that Dad was mobile and walked most places with his cane, so that wouldn't be necessary. I was then concerned about having the slacks cleaned which they assured me would be done properly by the in-house laundry...

214

…and that's another thing. There were times when I couldn't find a shirt for him that I knew he liked to wear, but rather found shirts with the names of other residents hanging in his closet. When I asked about that, and went to look for his shirt, I was told that a lot of the workers were foreign and didn't read English. Each time we visited him there was one more thing to sort out or look after for him. It made us really feel sorry for those who don't have any family coming by on a regular basis.

I could feel myself getting ready to investigate options for him, as we had for them, as a couple, in the Aspen Lodge. Firstly, the unit they had him in was a lockdown for mentally challenged residents. Having a meal with Dad meant listening to a man yell, groan, and otherwise make strange noises and arm gestures at the table. There was no one to chat with, which Dad was used to doing at meals. He wasn't totally keen on the food but appeared too polite to ask for anything else. I had told the staff that he usually had peanut butter and honey on his toast after his porridge. Each time I went I had to go and ask for it. They had it, but no one was paying any attention to this one resident's preferences, even though they assured us those kinds of things were part of the 'normal' services when we applied.

Because I had signed off on his medical treatment it took a few visits with the resident's doctor to feel like she understood where I was coming from and the responsibility I had taken for almost twenty years with Mom and Dad's medical issues. At one point the doctor asked me if Dad had any heart conditions and I said no. His heart and lungs had always tested great for his age and stage. She said she was concerned about his heart, because when she listened to it, something wasn't quite right. She also asked about putting Dad on antidepressants, but I didn't encourage that because we had seen a lot of seniors drugged to the point of being in a stupor even though they were dressed and strapped into their wheelchairs outside their rooms. I was so worried they would do that to him, and we felt he had more life in him than was being recognized or allowed at the facility.

We had two major issues and the first one was that none of the nurses or staff knew how to change Dad's ileostomy bag. We showed them how, each one as they came on duty when we were there and told them it was critical that it was emptied and cleaned every five hours. They arranged for the hospital to send down someone to give them a lesson, but we knew from how often they were running out of supplies that something wasn't right.

Dad also needed a proper bath once a week and that was also when the port that attached the ileostomy bag to his body was changed. The skin under the stoma needed to be cleaned and exposed to air for a bit. I was able to hire Erin once a week to bathe Dad and change his bag. That gave our family some peace of mind and gave Dad something good each week to look forward to. We were able to pay her from our family funds and it was well worth it. We couldn't depend on consistent care for this important condition by staff that had other duties and residents to look after.

Each step we took as things became evident made me more and more upset. We really thought that Dad would flourish without Mom because he was still so social. Putting him in that residence and having him in that lockdown unit with others who never engaged was terrible. It also didn't allow him to roam around and take advantage of some of the amenities that other residents did who were not in the lockdown unit. I often wondered if Dad was just assigned that room because it was the first vacant one after our application. It didn't suit his abilities or his personality.

Done With Dementia

Some of the nurses found out that he was a pastor and they would come around his bed, join hands and ask him to pray for them, which he was happy to do. They seemed to genuinely care for him. They told us they would come down to visit him during their breaks. But they also told us that every time they came into the room, he would be lying in the bed weeping as he looked up at the enlarged portrait of Mom made for her memorial service. They tried to comfort him. He wasn't paying any attention to the schedule, so they were sent down to bring him for meal time or a program in the common room. They also said that most of the time he just went to his bed and was sleeping or lying there. He didn't watch his TV. He didn't read any of the books we had left or his favorite magazines. He didn't watch any of the inspirational music videos and didn't answer either his landline, or his cell phone, both of which we had arranged for him.

For me personally it was awful because he was clear across a busy city that crossed two rivers with congested bridges and took me three times as long to get there compared to the house we had rented. Parking space at the complex was congested and we had to pay for it. I arranged parking passes for all of us in the family for extra convenience. Taking him anywhere was a real chore since it wasn't convenient to park, even for a few minutes, at the front curb. We had to navigate halls with lockdown doors, find him in his room, make sure he had the right clothes to go out and then get him into the car.

In addition to that, where he was located wasn't close to any of his favorite coffee shops or restaurants. The closest one was a little coffee kiosk in a gas station, so at least we could get him a treat and go for a little drive with it.

Linda McKendry

A week or so earlier I arranged to take him out of town to the hospital where his sister was. She had been in for a while and they were advising her family to come for final visits. I was having difficulty helping Dad in and out of the car. He seemed to need more help and I was a little annoyed with him for not cooperating with me more. We had such a good time in the hospital with his sister. Even though she was very sick, she was alert and coherent. My cousin, visiting his mother from down East, shared with me that it was my parents who had led him to faith in Christ at a time when he had a lot of doubts. That was news to me, but I was happy to know that.

I had asked my brother to come down to Calgary and take Dad for a little outing. Gary lived about one hour away and I knew he could handle helping Dad better than I had done when we went to visit Aunt Ferrell. Gary noticed that Dad was acting like he was in pain, but not saying too much. The reason became obvious the next morning. I got a call from one of the nurses that there was fresh blood in Dad's ileostomy bag. We had been warned that this was one of the symptoms that would mean an emergency. I asked the nurse to let me talk to Dad. I said, "Dad how are you feeling?" He said, "Not so good." I said, "Would you like to go to the hospital?" and he said, "No." In a flash I decided he wasn't going to go.... I said, "Ok. You don't have to. Just rest. Let me speak to the nurse again." I told the nurse that we weren't going to make him go through all that harangue of the ambulance and all that I knew he would have to endure... including emergency surgery... and for what? To come back there and live like he was?

I told her they could start palliative care and she said she would call the doctor. I sat back and took a deep breath. I knew full well what I had just said. I had witnessed my father-in-law in palliative care when he passed away and I knew how the process worked.

Done With Dementia

We had wanted to do palliative care with Mom and have her die at home, but when we found out that we would have to administer the medication, we opted out. Fortunately, she passed away before they could move her to a ward from the ICU or find a Hospice. God took care of that too.

I suddenly realized that my Dad's days, or hours, were numbered. I began to call the family to invite them to come and begin a bedside vigil after I explained my decision. I then realized I needed to get to my father's bedside and ask his forgiveness for being so mean to him where Mom was concerned. I would get frustrated at how he would treat Mom and I was mean with him about that. I didn't want him to go to his grave without giving myself a chance to confess and repent.

I told my husband what I had to do and that I was going over right away. He had an appointment at noon the same day at the hospital where he was having a pre-op for heart surgery. I called to let the staff tell Dad I would be there by 9:00 am. When we walked into the room Dad was lying in his bed. It was all neat and tidy, pulled up under his arms. His hands were folded on his chest and his eyes were closed. I immediately went over to his bed and kissed his cheek and reassured him that family were coming over to visit him. Then I knelt by his bed and told him how sorry I was for how I had treated him when I was mean. I asked him to forgive me. He didn't open his eyes. But he lifted his one arm closest to me and said, "I forgive you." I was weeping with relief but grieving at the same time.

I called their pastor, whose church Dad had founded over twenty-five years earlier. He was on his way. I also called Kim, who was taking her daughter Nicole to a quick orthodontist checkup. She said she would put Nicole's dance shoes and the tape recorder in the car and come over to do an Irish dance for Grandpa to cheer him up.

The pastor, Murray Swalm, arrived soon and greeted Dad. He nodded with a little smile, but once again he didn't open his eyes. When Murray asked Dad if he had a favorite portion of scripture, he said, "John 3:16." I was surprised because whenever I went with Dad as a girl to do hospital or home visits for the sick and shut-ins, he would always read Psalms 23. When Murray had to leave because of another commitment, and said goodbye to Dad, again he nodded in acknowledgment, but didn't open his eyes or say anything.

Soon after that Kim and Nicole arrived and when Dad heard the Irish tune, we noticed that one toe under the blanket was moving back and forth in time to the beat. He didn't open his eyes to watch her and she did two dances for him, but we were encouraged by that little movement that he was still with us in person and able to respond a little. Kim drew a chair by his side and when she noticed that he was cold, she reached into the closet and got out his favorite sweater that Mom had knit for him many years ago. She just laid it across his chest and over his shoulders. Again, he just nodded.

The staff in the facility brought down a cart with fresh coffee, cream, sugar, and muffins for the family, which I really appreciated. This was followed by the palliative care nurse who asked everyone to leave the room while she examined Dad. She came out with a little smile on her face. She said that when she lifted the covers to examine the condition of the skin on his legs, he said, "Your hands are cold!" She said, "So are yours." She then told me that his systems were shutting down and that she was ordering an increase in the prescribed palliative medication. She gave me some brochures to assist our family with the inevitable and explained that his body wouldn't be moved if he passed away before the other residents were in their rooms for the night.

She also told us that we were welcome to have as many family and friends come as we wanted and to feel free to use the seating area just outside the room too. It felt like the first time our needs were being considered without undue regard for all the other things. It helped that Dad's room was at the end of the hall and furthest away from the main meeting and eating areas.

The time came when Jim had to go for his pre-op appointment and as I bent over to give Dad a kiss, I heard myself saying, "Bye Dad!" instead of, "See you later!" which is what I usually said. His skin was very cold and clammy. He didn't open his eyes or move but he raised one hand in a little gesture of a wave. I knew that I might never see him again and it was hard to leave. It was great comfort to welcome Eldon who had just arrived and to know that Kim and Nicole were there with him too.

My other brother Gary and his wife Janice were on their way from their farm. Since Gary had driven up the evening before to take Dad out, as I had asked, I felt a little bad that he was turning around to make the trip again so soon, but I knew he was happy to come as soon as he could. Susie and Terry cut short their holiday in the States and were flying back. She was hoping that Dad would hang in there when he knew she was on her way. Eldon did his best to convey that to Dad. He nodded but didn't say anything, I was in the waiting room at the hospital while Jim filled out the necessary medical forms for his pre-op exam when my cell phone rang. It was about twenty minutes after twelve. It was my daughter. Her words were, "Grandpa's gone." I asked her when and she said, "A few minutes ago. Eldon and I were just here by his bed and he took his last breath and that was it. Are you going to be okay Mom?" I said, "Yes honey. I'll be fine." And as she hung up, I let out an uncontrolled sob and burst into tears. I tried to compose myself by telling the waiting room patients that my Dad just died.

God arranged for me to be sitting next to a large woman, dressed in a Hawaiian Mumu with big wavy hair and a big necklace. She immediately held me close to her chest and hugged me. She handed me a tissue to blow my nose just as Jim was called into his appointment. It seemed so strange to just get up and follow him and a nurse down a cold strange hall and have to switch gears in my mind to be in the present; to be a supportive wife. When we got into the examining room, I immediately told the nurse, "My Dad just died." She said she was sorry to hear that and the doctor would be right in. I realized that in a hospital you might hear those words often and they wouldn't mean much. It took everything I had to stay calm and be attentive towards Jim's situation. I would cry later!

I decided then and there I didn't want to go back to CB. I didn't want to see Dad's body. I wanted to remember him like I had seen him last. I called Eldon who was still there and asked him if he and Gary could pack up the room of Dad's stuff and put out the clothes they decided he would be buried in. His black slacks with the suspenders. The white shirt. The green jacket which he loved because it was "Irish". I asked that they include his shamrock encrusted pen that he used for doing his word search puzzles and a necktie… Dad always wore a tie if he wore a jacket.

It was such a relief to have responsible, loving brothers to give that job to. They had to drive to our house to pick up the boxes, but everything was there because the move into CB was so recent. I counted the days from when Mom had died, and it was 69 days! Barely over two months. The doctor said he died of "heart congestion" or as I called it, "A broken heart." I believe that if one of us had been willing to take him in regardless and have family around with more familiar things he might have thrived a little longer.

Dad died just a little before Aunt Farrell. As it turned out, Dad's memorial service was planned on a Sunday, after church on St. Patrick's Day in 2013, and Aunt Ferrell's was the day before. I felt God arranged this so the many relatives that came from all over got a "two for one" that weekend! I knew Dad was looking down over the balconies of heaven watching us memorialize his life in a place where he had so many friends and family. It was a good ending. Good closure.

Life has a way of only teaching us as we go along, and we seem to have to make some decisions and go down the road a bit in order to know whether it's the right way or not. In some cases, we can backtrack, or take a new road to a better place. In Dad's case we were still full of hope that we could find the solution to his circumstances and give him a life worth living.

Susie had stopped in to visit Dad once when they were having a hymn sing in the common room. She was playing the piano and they didn't want her to stop. She said that was the happiest she ever saw Dad at the CB. It's because he was engaging with others in fellowship and doing something he had his heart in. It was lively and inspiring after which he had to go back to a lonely room and face the portrait on the wall of his beloved Lydia. I was glad that God had taken him home. He didn't suffer and I didn't put him through modern life-saving techniques in a noisy hospital setting just to prolong his life, and for what? He died peacefully as

Linda McKendry

one of four generations in the room. We sent him home to Lydia, the love of his life, next to Jesus, his Savior.

We believed that Mom was asking everyone in heaven, "Where's my Johnny?" and God finally had to bring him home to be with her and keep them together. Believing in heaven as our final and eternal resting place when we die gives us so much hope and joy that they are in a better place. And guess what else? They are definitely and finally DONE-WITH-DEMENTIA!

The Big Promise Kept with Some Regrets

This time we didn't have to worry about keeping them together here on earth. God took care of that when he took them home. We had the idea that if Dad passed away before Mom, she wouldn't survive for long. But we also thought that if Mom passed away before Dad, he would do fine. He was mobile, alert, and still very sociable.

Regrets Looking Back:

Many times, when we express regret, people will ask, "What would you have done differently, knowing what you know now?" I can't change the past but if you are using our story to decide if you CAN or WANT to keep your parents together my regrets might help.

My regrets are from what we found out after the fact. The first one was regretting that the transition into the Assisted Living couldn't be honored once the house was emptied and sold.

They couldn't come back to their own home if it wasn't working out. Susie and I felt that we had not kept that part of the promise to them. However, if we had done that, would they have spent more time over at the house, just back in the same situation as before? Obviously without the main pieces of furniture they needed they would have had to go back to the Aspen each night at least. And they would have had their meals there if they remembered in time to get there.

That may have been more confusing for them. I don't have any regrets for taking them out of the Assisted Living. I'm glad I didn't leave them there so long that a crisis would have separated them, and we would have had different things to deal with. If one of them had been sent to the hospital from the Lodge, how much authority would I have had at that point? The system can sometimes kick in automatically and you are left with finding out what to do, who to contact, and what the process is as it happens. Several times when Dad was in hospital approaching the ten days, there was a social worker there to make arrangements to send him to a facility if he didn't have adequate home care. The fact that we had more than enough, including qualified live-in nurses and around the clock care, gave them the confidence to release our parent back to us.

Another regret I have, again with no way to prove anything different, is when I sent them away and we cleaned out their rooms at the Lodge. When they came home, they came to a strange place. When I picture what it would have been like to have them there, I know they would have been just sitting close by and watching the whole procedure. I can't believe Mom would know what was going on, but if Dad was all right, she would have been fine. I couldn't have anticipated the sewer back up on their first night in their new home. I regret that I didn't stay overnight the first week or so.

Linda McKendry

I made assumptions that having my office combined with their new home would work as a win-win for both of us. Again because of dementia, that was not the case, but thankfully, we were able to make the necessary adjustments and put the right things in order.

I have absolutely no regrets over taking the responsibility to care for them and find the answers to any problem that might arise. It was easy to tell people, "Left to the system they wouldn't be together and wouldn't have the lifestyle they like best." That was it in a nutshell. And having them in Assisted Living for the seven months proved enough that we didn't have to fight with the system to keep them together. In fact, we were rewarded with the funding to make it a little easier.

Looking back, we didn't take into consideration the grieving process of losing your wife after 65 years of marriage. We learned so much about how the professional facilities for seniors work, with both at the Lodge, and with Dad at the CB. I know I would have taken Dad out of there too, given more time. I would have figured out a way. We counted on having him spend up to three months with each one of us kids. I believe that may have helped him to feel less lonely and abandoned. We went from being there 24/7 to only seeing him a few times a week. I was in the middle of my husband's medical crisis and many times wishing Dad was living in our home so I could look after both without so much time wasted driving.

Conclusion: We put, "Only 69 Days Apart" on their grave marker. The last five years, from spring 2008 to spring 2013 were a 24/7 commitment. I often tell people that the saving grace for me was that both didn't have a medical crisis at the same time! We were only doing extra time in hospital or with diagnosis and treatments with one while the other was stable and usually in tow. Mostly still together. Mom is now with her Johnny for eternity and we know they are totally Done-With-Dementia.

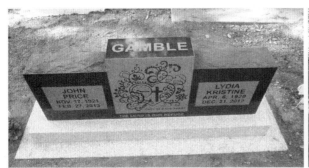 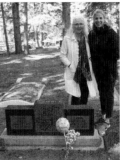

Bless you as you make the most Legal, Logical, and Loving
decisions on behalf of your parents.
Keep them together if you can and remember
what they need most is each other.

GALLERY

About Mom (Lydia Kristine) from Her Memorial Service Brochure

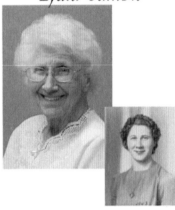

Lydia Gamble

Woman of God, Sister
Wife, Mother, Grandmother
Great-grandmother, Friend
Missionary & Mentor

April 6th, 1920 - December 21, 2012

Be at peace again, my soul, for the Lord
has done good things for you.
Psalm 116:7

Loved, Cherished,
& Honored

My Story...

Parents were Alida and Peter
Tiessen, who eventually
settled north of Drumheller
on a farm. They worked
very hard as immigrant
settlers and Lydia had to
learn to do a lot of chores,
both inside and out. Her
father influenced her musical
talents and they used to play
duets on the same guitar!
Her mother was a master at
working with animals but
could also cook, sew, and
managed to find lace for
curtains and trim on home
made dresses.

Born on April 6th, 1920,
in Arkadak, Russia, her
original name was Lieda
Tiessen, with her full
name shown as Lydia
Kristine on the certificate
of Canadian Citizenship.

Lydia &
brother Alfred

Sister Ruthie

...the early years...

Lydia went to grade school at the one room school house
across the road from their farm. As she became one of the
older students, she worked at the school cleaning, keeping
the fires stoked, and fetching water. Rural life was always
busy with chores and hard work, but fun was found in
winter sports: skating on the creek, skiing on barrel staves
strapped to their boots behind a horse, and making music
inside. Summer was helping with the garden, including
enjoying her favorite flowers: pansies and sweet peas.

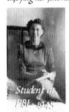

Student in
PBI - 1945

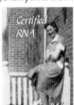

Certified
RNA

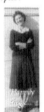

Happily
Single

...enter Mr. Right

...and starting a family...

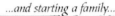

Married
Rev John Gamble

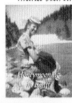
Honeymooning
in Banff

Ellon

Li

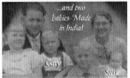
...and two
babies "Made
in India!
Gary

Suzi

India meant language school and servants and saying good bye to kids as they went off to boarding school. It was serving her Lord and using every gift and talent she was blessed with.

...and just being a good wife, mother, grandmother, great-grandmother & friend...

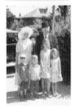
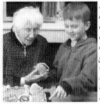

She saw each of her kids at least once a month and often four generations in one place! Always a loving hand to hold.

...leisure activities in later years...

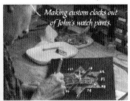
Making custom clocks out of John's watch parts.

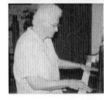

Reading and hand crafts were enjoyed less and less as the motivation and memory decreased. However, up to the very week she passed away she was still sitting at the piano and playing 'It Will Be Worth It All' and 'I've Got a Mansion' with natural flow.

...fun outings and events...

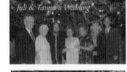
Juli & Tanner's Wedding

Banff a favorite

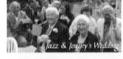
Jazz & Jenny's Wedding

Memorial Day

Train to B.C.

Kid's School Picnic

Ft. Langley Festival

Keenagers

Boating

Parades

...side by side...

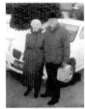

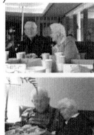

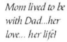

Mom lived to be with Dad...her love... her life!

In April 2008, the children took Mom and Dad out of assisted living and leased a bungalow for them to call home. Left to the system they would not have remained together as a couple, and their quality of life would not have included their favorite activities, music, and treats.

For Mom that meant being with Dad. For us it meant commitments to round the clock care with help from Self Managed Care Funding..

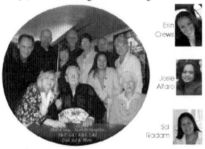

Erin Crews

Josie Alfaro

Sol Radam

Special Tribute to the following:
Surgeon: Dr. Blue, Foothill Hospital
Gastologist: Dr. Adrienne Cohen
Pharmacist: David @ Blue Bottle
Dentists: Dr. Willy & Heinz Dyck
Denturist: Dr. Ken Moore
Hairdresser: Gina @ Foxy Locks

Pediculist: Noorani
Family Doctors:
 Dr. Terry Unger
 Dr. Ken Yee (retired)
 Dr. Marianne Botha
Hired Caregivers: Sol, Fabienne, Rachel, Josie, & Erin

MEMORIAL SERVICE FOR LYDIA KRISTINE GAMBLE

January 5th, 2013
Bergen, Alberta, Canada

Officiating: Rev. Willard Swalm

Prelude: Lydia's Favorite Hymns
Opening Remarks & Prayer
Obituary
Hymn: In the Garden
Journal Reading - Linda McKendry
Hymn: I've Got a Mansion
Slide Presentation
Eulogy- Gary Gamble
Message: Pastor David Benjamin
Closing Remarks & Prayer

NOTE: Reception to follow in adjacent area.

I've Got A Mansion

I'm satisfied with just a cottage below
A little silver and a little gold
But in that city where the ransomed will shine
I want a gold one that's silver lined

I've got a mansion just over the hilltop
In that bright land where we'll never grow old
And some day yonder we will never more wander
But walk on streets that are purest gold

Don't think me poor or deserted or lonely
I'm not discouraged I'm heaven bound
I'm but a pilgrim in search of the city
I want a mansion, a harp and a crown

I've got a mansion just over the hilltop
In that bright land where we'll never grow old
And some day yonder we will never more wander
But walk on streets that are purest gold

It Will Be Worth It All

Sometimes the day seems long,
Our trials hard to bear.
We're tempted to complain,
to murmur and despair.
But Christ will soon appear
to catch his bride away!
All tears forever over
in God's eternal day!

CHORUS:
It will be worth it all
when we see Jesus!
Life's trials will seem so small
when we see Christ.
One glimpse of his dear face,
all sorrow will erase.
So, bravely run the race
till we see Christ.

At times the sky seems dark,
with not a ray of light;
We're tossed and driven on,
no human help in sight.
But there is One in heaven,
Who knows our deepest care;
Let Jesus solve your problems,
just go to him in prayer.

Life's day will soon be o're,
all storms forever past;
We'll cross the great divide
to Glory, safe at last!
We'll share the joys of heaven:
a harp, a home, a crown;
The tempter will be banished,
We'll lay our burdens down.

About Dad (John Price) from His Memorial Service Brochure

Rev. John Gamble

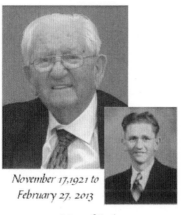

November 17, 1921 to
February 27, 2013

Man of God
Merchant Marine
Minister & Missionary
Master of Clock and Watch Repair

*Be at peace again, my soul, for the Lord
has done good things for you.*
Psalm 116:7

God is our refuge and strength...
Psalm 46:1a

Loved, Cherished,
& Honored

My Story...

Parents were Ira Samuel Gamble, born in Missouri, USA and Anna Estella Harvey, born in Kansas, USA. Both were school teachers with 14 years difference in their age.

They immigrated to Canada in the early 1800's and eventually settled as pioneers in the Niche Valley south of Sundre, Alberta.

They had twelve children and left a legacy of God fearing heirs with a strong work ethic and compassion for others less fortunate.

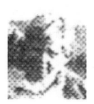

Born on November 17th, 1921, in Niche Valley, south of Sundre, Alberta, John Price Gamble was the sixth child. Three older sisters were there to see that he stayed out of trouble. Two older brothers passed down shoes, shirts & pants.

Early years were filled with many farm chores and family prayer times that included great singing.

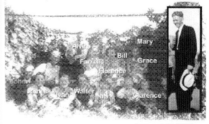

Mary
Bill
Grace
Florence
Clarence
Walter

...the Merchant Marine....

Wanting to serve his country during the World War II as a Conscientious Objector, who wouldn't bear arms, he saw an ad for "Marine Engineer". He trained in Prescott, Ontario before being assigned to the USS Banff merchant supply ship shovelling coal. India was one of the countries visited during this duty and that is when John felt the call of God to give his life to serve the people of that country.

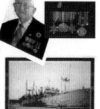

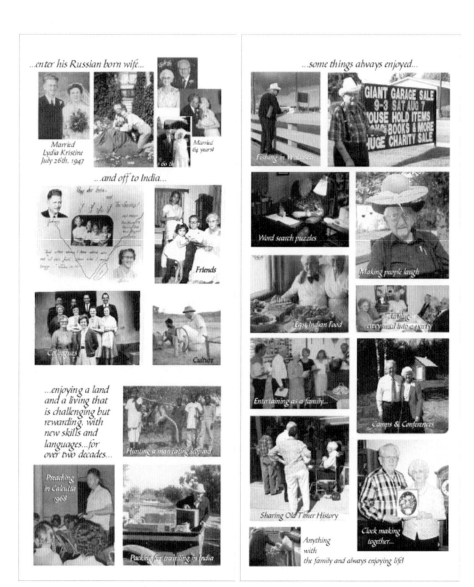

...enter his Russian born wife...

Married
Lydia Kristine
July 26th, 1947

56th

Married
65 years!

60 th

...and off to India...

Friends

Colleagues

Culture

...enjoying a land
and a living that
is challenging but
rewarding, with
new skills and
languages...for
over two decades...

Hunting a man eating leopard

Preaching
in Calcutta
1968

Packing for travelling in India

...some things always enjoyed...

GIANT GARAGE SALE
9-3 SAT AUG 7
HOUSE HOLD ITEMS
BOOKS & MORE
HUGE CHARITY SALE

Fishing in Waboose

Word search puzzles

Making people laugh

East Indian Food

Turning
everyone into a party

Entertaining as a family...

Camps & Conferences

Sharing Old Timer History

Clock making
together...

Anything
with
the family and always enjoying life!

232

...side by side...

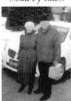

They only had 69 days apart. Mom went on to heaven Dec. 21.2012. Laid to rest on January 4th, 2013.

In April 2008, the children took Mom and Dad out of assisted living and leased a bungalow for them to call home. Left to the system they would not have remained together as a couple, and their quality of life would not have included their favorite activities, music, and treats.

For Mom that meant being with Dad. For us it meant commitments to round the clock care with help from Self Managed Care Funding..

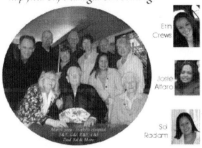

Erin Crews

Josie Alfaro

Sol Radam

Special Tribute to the following:
Surgeon: Dr. Buie, Foothill Hospital
Gerfologist: Dr. Adrienne Cohen
Dentists: Drs. Heinz and Willy Dyck
Pharmacist: David @ Blue Bottle
Calgary Hearing Clinic
Pedicurist: Noorani

Family Doctors:
Dr. Terry Unger
Dr. Ken Yee (retired)
Dr. Marianne Botha
Hired Caregivers: Sol, Fabienne, Rachel, Josie, & Erin
Staff at Colonel Belcher Carewest

MEMORIAL SERVICE FOR REV. JOHN P. GAMBLE

March 17th, 2013
Calgary, Alberta, Canada
Officiating: Rev. Murray Swarm

Prelude..................................Family's Favorite Hymns
Welcome & Prayer...........................Pastor Murray

Doxology

Obituary...Harvey Gamble

Song
Where Can I Go But To The Lord

Slide Presentation............................*The Man of God*
Eulogy...Eldon Gamble

Personal Comments:

Iris Baker	*The Missionary*
Solo	'Thank You' ....Penny Gamble
Sam & Brenda Lachman	*The Minister & Friend*
Don Bradshaw	*The Clock & Watch Maker*

Presentation to Bonavista Church
Message of Comfort ....Pastor Murray
Closing Prayer & Benediction

Irish Dance: Nicole Hounsome
Reception in Foyer

Four Generations Present as Dad Stepped into Eternity...

Dad was Irish and proud of it. He used to tell Lab technicians that he had "green Irish blood". He was laid to rest in his green jacket with a favorite shamrock encrusted pen he used for word search puzzles. It's Providence that picked St. Patrick's day to share his life and legacy.

Family members were notified of Dad's condition and asked to come and stay with him. Eldon, the oldest son, arrived first. Others came and went. His grand-daughter, Kim, and his great-grand-daughter, Nicole, on their way from an appointment came by. They brought Nicole's dance shoes and an Irish folk music CD to cheer him up.

She was born with a rare condition that causes the joints in her legs and hips to be so painful it can be immobilizing. So for her to want to take up Irish Dance and win medals is nothing short of a miracle. She didn't see her great grandpa do an Irish jig and scare the physio therapist, but she did hear his feet tapping under the lunch table a few times..

Little did they know that within minutes of her simple recital at his bedside he would enter eternity so peacefully with just the four of them there. Dad, Eldon, Kim, and Nicole.
One from each generation!

Together to the End… the last five years

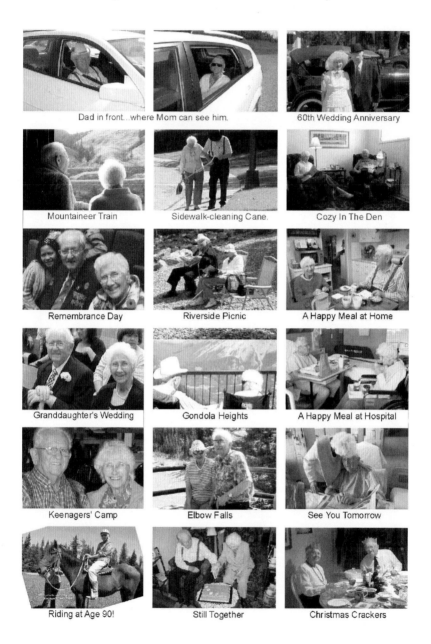

Dad in front…where Mom can see him.

60th Wedding Anniversary

Mountaineer Train

Sidewalk-cleaning Cane.

Cozy In The Den

Remembrance Day

Riverside Picnic

A Happy Meal at Home

Granddaughter's Wedding

Gondola Heights

A Happy Meal at Hospital

Keenagers' Camp

Elbow Falls

See You Tomorrow

Riding at Age 90!

Still Together

Christmas Crackers

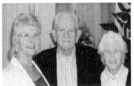

Easter After the Lodge

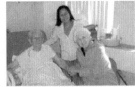

Visiting Dad Twice a Day

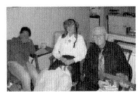

Christmas Comedy

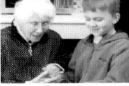

Great Grandson Near

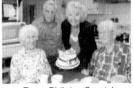

Every Birthday Special

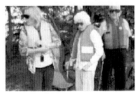

Riverboat Tour

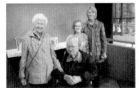

Great Grand daughter's Art

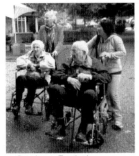

Cranberry Festival

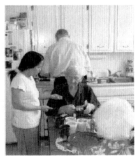

Home Care Recovery

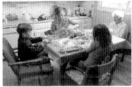

Great Grandchildren's Fun

GIVING LIFE TO THE FULLEST FOR FAMILY

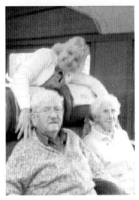

A Train Adventure

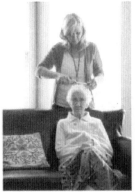

Best Hairdresser

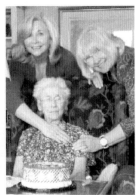

All Done With Love!

DECIDING IF YOU CAN OR WANT TO DO WHAT WE DID

Survey: What You need to KNOW...

What You Need to Know About Your Parents

If you have lived with or near your parents for many years, you will automatically know a lot about them. You may have sat and told stories to each other and recounted memories from your childhood. In the process you find out a lot about their guiding principles, ideologies, habits, routines and what their preferences are. How they got through the tough times tells you a lot about them too. However, if dementia is creeping in and memory is failing, what you can recall becomes very important to them. Here is a survey to help you make your list.

PAST

What have they always done: habits, routines, and traditions?

What are their likes and dislikes? Make a list of:

- Friends and Family
- Food and Favorite Eating Places
- Clothing and Styles
- Home Décor and Environment
- People and Professionals They Know
- Music and Entertainment

- Leisure and Hobbies
- Other interests, such as clubs, memberships, and religious traditions.

PRESENT

It's more important to look at your parents' current condition to assess urgent needs. Get help from local home care and medical professionals if there are issues you can't describe. These include:

- Mental State, Mind Set and General Mood
- Ability to Perform Usual Tasks
- Mobility and Balance
- Energy and Strength Levels
- Sleep Patterns
- Finances, Debt, Bill Payment Process
- Medical Conditions and Prescriptions
- Other Challenges and Obvious Changes

Avoid making them feel like you are interrogating them. Set aside a good time to be with them. An overnight stay, if possible, or an offer to take them for an outing or a short trip will give you an opportunity to see if there are things they are struggling with.

Many of us are in denial and don't want to face the need for hearing aids, canes, or walkers. We want to feel youthful and strong. We want to keep doing what we have always done. Your parents are no different.

Check around the house and see if things are piling up, not being stored properly, or in need of repair or cleaning. These will all be signs that they need some help. They may be very proud and since they are the parents, they may not want to burden you with their issues.

Check out resources online that will help you figure out the best ways to approach them about these things. One of the most sensitive issues is money. Utility and credit card statements are good signs that the routine expenses are being taken care of.

Don't be afraid to ask the hard questions prefaced by letting them know you are eager to make sure their wishes for their future are taken care of. They will need to be reminded that if, God forbid, dementia should strike, or either of them should have an accident, don't they want to know someone they love, and trust is looking out for their best interests?

If they won't open up to you, ask them if there is someone they prefer, a close friend or a sibling to have a frank discussion with. Someone else in the family may have more information. It doesn't hurt to have "family meetings" and include everyone in the discussions. You are welcome to use my book, my course, or other materials and referred services to help in this important fact-finding mission.

If you wait, it could be too late.

If they are in reasonable health, you can begin by dropping by on occasion and doing little things around the house to help out. My brothers and I came to our parents' home once and helped Dad clean out the garage. We had noticed Dad's garage was becoming a hazard with too much stuff accumulating in it. We sat him on a stool with a calendar and a clip board to make notes while we sorted through stuff. We got his opinion on each item to store, fix, give away, or trash. Mom came out with a tray of coffee and cookies. It was fun and very productive. Sorting through nuts, bolts, nails, screws, washers and putting them into clear containers not only saved him time and money,but it made downsizing a lot easier when we ultimately helped them with that. They will "test before they trust." And you want to pass the test.

FUTURE

Know their thoughts about the future. Dad had chosen the Aspen Lodge Assisted Living facility because he regularly did chaplain services there. A couple of his parishioners lived there and gave glowing reports about the facility. We knew they wanted to stay in their own home if possible, but they found some of the home maintenance issues challenging as I have shared.

Some medical conditions are progressive, so you have a good idea from the medical diagnosis and prognosis what to expect sooner or later. Here are some of the most important things to plan for:

- Legal Documents
- Will. Personal Directive. EPOA
- Living Arrangements
- Home Care
- Assisted Living
- Downsizing
- Medical Needs
- Finances

You can use the surveys included in this book or downloaded from the website to give you guidance.

WORST CASE SCENARIO

People often complain when I mention planning for the worst. They say it's "fear mongering" or "being negative". But I found that thinking about the worst that could happen helped me to be prepared, if not in reality, then at least in my mind. What would I need? What action might I have to take?

For example, when I thought that both of them might be bedridden with severe mental and or medical conditions I imagined the living room with two hospital beds. I knew there was

Linda McKendry

equipment available to help lift patients. I also believed that the same medications given in facilities would be available to us and we already had certified nurses to administer those. I pictured them able to either see each other and to hold hands because of what we could put in place. Just having that picture in my mind gave my heart comfort and strength to carry on.

Here's my list of "What ifs...."

- ACCIDENT affecting
- Body

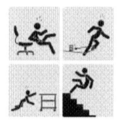

- Mobility
- Discomfort (pain)
- Brain

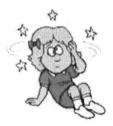

- Mental State
- Memory
- Mood

DISEASE

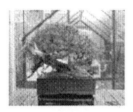

- Debilitating
- Untreatable
- Terminal

FINANCES

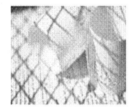

- Unknown
- Inaccessible
- Out of Control
- Insufficient

FACILITY

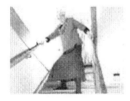

- Unsuitable
- Unavailable
- Unaffordable
- None available

Linda McKendry

CARE

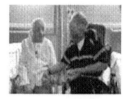

- Unknown
- Unavailable
- Unsuitable

Put all of these together...

- <u>Asking</u> some tough questions allows you to ensure they aren't just saying they are ahead of the game when they might not be. Dad thought he had things in place, but many documents had to be upgraded, modified, or revisited from years ago.
- <u>Ignoring the Topic. Don't Want to Discuss.</u> This is the greatest challenge. Do what you can and keep in mind it's hard for many parents to admit they need help. Especially from their children.
- More Desperate Than Anyone Realized.
- <u>Victims of Dementia?</u> No One Guessed? <u>If</u> it isn't too severe you can still visit a lawyer or their doctor to determine if they can sign off on choosing their EPOA.

There are legal ways for the court to appoint you to take over their affairs if you are willing to do that and can afford the legal fees.

Just being the "next of kin" and particularly one of the children will get you through a lot of doors on their behalf.

- <u>Don't Know Where to Turn for Help.</u> Your parents may know they need help but didn't realize they could turn to you or anyone else for help.
- There are lots of programs available if you know where to look and who to ask. Most require application or professional referrals.
- <u>Relieved That You Have Shown Up!</u> If this describes your parents, take it to heart and be happy.

IT'S YOUR DECISION

I want you to answer this right now but wait to make your final decision. I want you to be confident that this is something you CAN and WANT to do. That way you will take the challenge with commitment.

- I CAN see myself contributing to their care.
- Help with Preparation and Plans
- Part Time
- Full Time
- I CAN'T see myself contributing to their care.
- I DON'T WANT TO contribute to their care.
- Honest
- Realistic
- Love 'n Prayer… go a long way too!

Take the next step: GO RESEARCH OPTIONS

Even if you feel it's all so overwhelming and you don't want to contribute to your parent's care on any level, please continue to search your heart and ask the hard questions.

Information is power, as they say, and when you see what we did and how we did it, you may change your mind, or share this with others who want to contribute to their parents' care. In any case, there is no pressure or guilt allowed! And no competition.

It's healthier all around to admit you don't want to, then to be pressured or guilted into such a huge responsibility.

God Bless You and Your Family,

Including Your Precious Parents!

ACKNOWLEDGEMENTS

My appreciation and gratitude go out to my brother Eldon (and his wife Ruth), my next brother Gary (and his wife Janice), and a very special thanks to my little sister, Esther Susan, affectionately called Susie (and her husband, Doctor Terry). Each of them came to our aid when called and all of us went above and beyond the call of duty to say that we have no regrets.

The VIPs in their life were their doctors and other professionals who had their best interests at heart. These are the people who gave good advice and took our opinions seriously because of the level of care we were administering.

The home care, live-in nurses, we hired were invaluable for their assistance and willingness to "perform other duties as required" for Mom and Dad, our family, friends and guests who visited them. They all went above and beyond the call of duty. Our boarder, Joe, falls into this category too for his offers to help and never complain.

My daughter Kim supported me in practical ways and her children were encouraged to enjoy their great grandparents which made being a family more fun. My husband was one of those who didn't get in or out, but did stay out of the way so I had the freedom to do what was required and still come home for respite.

Adria Laycraft, a freelance editor, edited my manuscripts, made good suggestions, and didn't slap my hands for the habit of two spaces after each sentence. As a relative, the story is more close to home and personal. info@adrialaycraft.com or
www. adrialaycraft.com

ABOUT THE AUTHOR

Linda McKendry (nee Gamble) is the firstborn daughter of John and Lydia Gamble. Her parents took her and her brother, Eldon, to India on their Missionary Assignment in 1952. She was educated in Woodstock International Boarding School in the Himalayas from Kindergarten through Grade Nine (American Curriculum). This made her a "child of the global village" and a "third world kid."

The two youngest siblings, Gary and Susie, were born in India, and all of them grew up with experiences of other nationalities, cultures, languages, and religions. Separate dorms, classes and nine months separation from their parents made family bonding weak. Working together to care for their parents brought them together in a very special way.

Linda is married to Jim and has two children, three stepchildren and five grandchildren. She lives in Calgary, Alberta, Canada.

Her career followed her talents and interest in art and music.

Interest in art led to a commercial art degree from Washington School of Art combined with Graphic Arts and Desktop Publishing courses. These skills were used for consulting, instructing, public speaking opportunities, and writing primarily for the Gift, Tableware, and Fashion industries.

Self-labelled "overqualified and undereducated" is a testament to a life lived with many interests and experience in a lot of fields. She has founded and run several businesses that changed as necessary based on husbands' corporate transfers. She's also had "real jobs" as an employee. She was once a "Display Manager and Advertising Coordinator" for Eaton's and another time became the first female sales rep for a 75-year-old distribution company, bringing a specialty fabrication system from Germany to Canada.

She educates, motivates, inspires, and entertains audiences and target markets in whatever topic or theme her clients need for their dealer networks. She also continues to help clients with leasehold improvement designs and plans as they increase and expand.

Like her father, she claims she's not "retired"... but "re-treaded!" Still going long and strong with God's help! Her calling in life is to take "people, places, and things" to their next level.

She hopes that readers will feel they are taken to their next level in understanding that a lot can be done-with-dementia to keep parents together.

You can find out more of her history and the corporations she has worked for at

www.visiquad.com and www.todaysdisplays.com.

Linda is working on Online Courses, Seminars, Workshops, and a Workbook.

www.done-with-dementia.com